STYLE AND SATIRE

FASHION IN PRINT

1777–1927

Catherine Flood and Sarah Grant

V&A Publishing

First published by V&A Publishing, 2014
Victoria and Albert Museum
South Kensington
London SW7 2RL
www.vandapublishing.com

Distributed in North America by
Harry N. Abrams Inc., New York

ISBN 978 1 85177 803 4

Library of Congress Control Number 2014932325

10 9 8 7 6 5 4 3 2 1
2018 2017 2016 2015 2014

A catalogue record for this book is available from the British Library.

Printed in China

V&A Publishing

Supporting the world's leading museum of art and design, the Victoria and Albert Museum, London

Every effort has been made to seek permission to reproduce those images whose copyright does not reside with the V&A, and we are grateful to the individuals and institutions who have assisted in this task. Any omissions are entirely unintentional, and the details should be addressed to V&A Publishing.

Designed by Emily Chicken, Peepstudio, with artworking by Lila Hamilton
New photography by Richard Davis and George Eksts, V&A Photographic Studio

Front cover: James Gillray (1756–1815), **'Characters in High Life. Sketch'd at the New Rooms, Opera House'** (detail, p.43)

Back cover: André Edouard Marty (1882–1974), **'Les Ailes Dans Le Vent'**, published in the *Modes et manières d'aujourd'hui*, Paris, 1919. National Art Library: 95.JJ.24

p.4: Georges Jacques Gatine (1773–c.1841), after Horace Vernet (1789–1863), **'Merveilleuse: Chapeau de paille d'Italie, par-dessus à la Chinoise.'** (Merveilleuse: Italian straw hat, overdress in the Chinese style.) (detail, p.53)

p.6: James Gillray (1756–1815), after an anonymous French print, **'Les Invisibles'** (detail, pp.46–7)

p.32: William Heath (1795–1840), **'La Poule. Quadrille – Evening Fashions – Dedicated to the HEADS of the Nation'** (detail, p.59)

p.76: J. Coventry (lithographer), **'Mrs Bloomer's Own'** (detail, p.60)

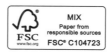

CONTENTS

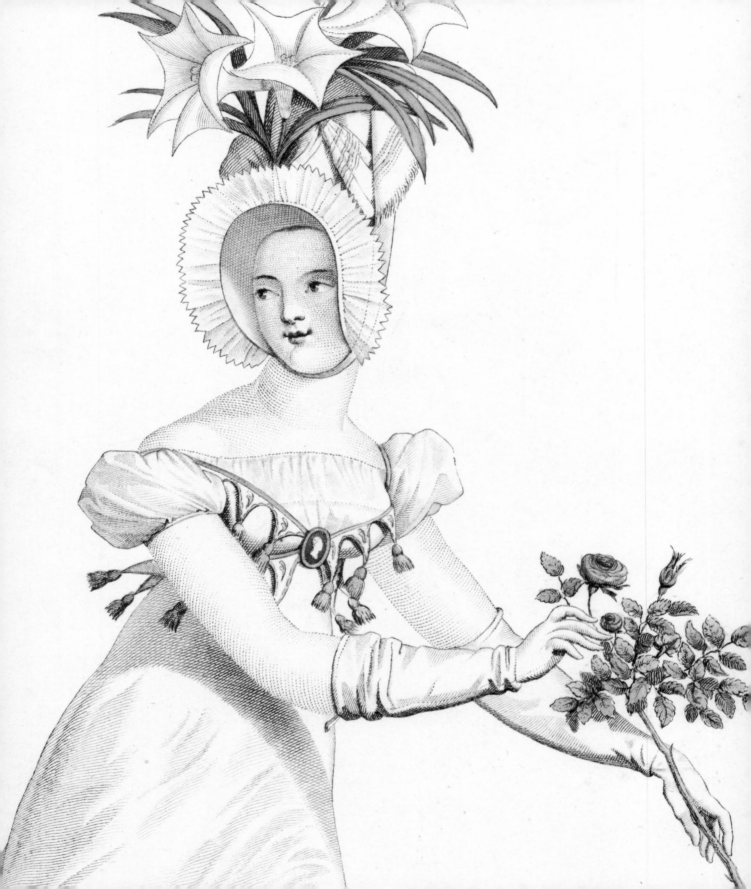

AUTHORS' NOTE

Style and Satire: Fashion in Print 1777–1927 reveals the close and previously little-studied connections between two forms of printed art: fashion plates – prints designed to serve as an appealing, detailed record of contemporary styles – and graphic social satire, by which we mean printed and drawn works of art that caricature social mores for humorous ends.[1] It draws largely on the Victoria and Albert Museum's holdings, in particular its collection of fashion plates, long recognized by scholars as one of the finest of its kind.[2] These are housed as loose prints in the Museum's Word & Image Department, and in bound volumes in the National Art Library at the V&A, South Kensington.

This book is not a chronological survey of the history of dress, nor the history of the print – complex subjects, for which a considerable wealth of literature already exists. Rather, it is an introduction to the links between those two art forms, exploring some of the most important themes connecting works that issued from Paris and London, the two centres of fashion and print culture in Europe, between the end of the eighteenth century and the beginning of the twentieth. We aim to provide a glimpse of the riches of the V&A's holdings, as well as increasing the reader's understanding and enjoyment of these beautiful prints.

Catherine Flood and Sarah Grant

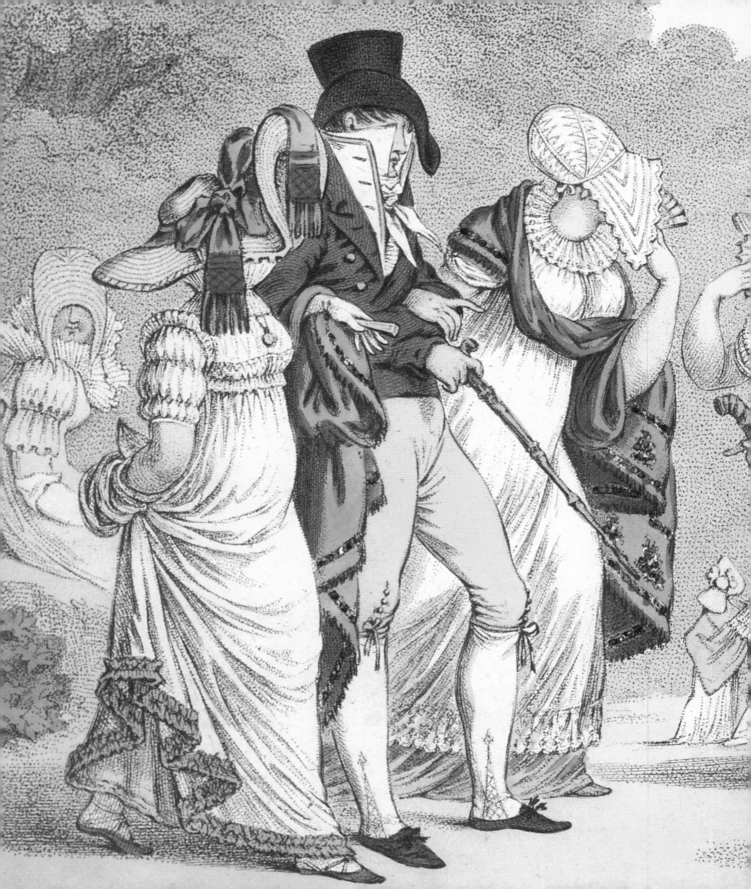

STYLE AND SATIRE: CREATING FASHION FANTASIES

Catherine Flood and Sarah Grant

Beautifully printed and hand-coloured fashion plates – artistically-realized prints illustrating aspects of contemporary dress and deportment – flourished in Europe from the late eighteenth century until the 1930s. They communicated trends in fashionable dress and provided readers with a fantasy of luxury and consumption. Over the same period, fashion was a regular target for satirists, who claimed to expose social truths through their humorously exaggerated depictions of already extreme styles. While fashion plates sold an ideal, satirical prints gloried in the absurdity of fashion, sometimes betraying darker social and moral anxieties. Fashion plates and fashion satires created opposing fantasies of fashion: the elegant and the grotesque, the refined and the repellent, the ideal and the imperfect. They were in reality, however, two sides of the same coin. Together, they helped to foster a culture of fashion; as Sharon Marcus points out: 'Fashion depends on quick dissemination in time and extensive distribution in space: a fashion is only one if many people simultaneously learn of it, adopt it and renounce it.'[1] In an industrialized, age the print market had an important role to play in fulfilling these requirements.

In his seminal 1864 essay on art and modernity, *The Painter of Modern Life*, the art critic and poet Charles Baudelaire (1821–67) singled out for attention fashion plates and magazine illustration, because they depicted everyday life at a time when academic art dealt almost exclusively with grand themes from history, religion and mythology. Indeed, the attention that Baudelaire pays to fashion plates and magazine illustration is then borne out by the influence they had on other forms concerned with representing contemporary life in the nineteenth century. Paul Cézanne (1839–1906), for example, is known to have copied a fashion plate in his painting *La Promenade* (*c*.1871). Valerie Steele suggests that the conventionalized

gestures found in fashion plates may well have seemed to Cézanne a more modern and relevant model than the classical sources employed by many of his peers.[2] Echoes of fashion plate compositions can also be discerned in the mannered poses of nineteenth-century *carte de visite* portraits (inexpensive, portable photographs), capturing sitters dressed in their best clothes. The humble fashion plate proved itself a useful template for picturing modern life, from modern art to photography.

Baudelaire's character, 'the painter of modern life', is a magazine illustrator (modelled on the French illustrator Constantin Guys, 1802–92), who wanders the streets, alive to the continuously changing city-as-spectacle:

> If in a shift of fashion, the cut of a dress has been slightly modified, if clusters of ribbons and curls have been dethroned by rosettes, if bonnets have widened and chignons have come down a little on the nape of the neck, if waistlines have been raised and skirts become fuller, you may be sure that from a long way off his eagle eye will have detected it.[3]

This he captures by 'the quickest and the cheapest technical means,' because 'there is in the trivial things of life, in the daily changing of external things, a speed of movement that imposes upon the artist an equal speed of execution.'[4] For Baudelaire, the subject matter of fashion and the ephemeral medium of printed illustration, together, captured the thrilling immediacy of his contemporary world.

The print was a tool as essential in early modern life as photographs and digital media are to us today; an urban and commercial phenomenon that was, for its time, comparatively democratic.[5] Fashion plates and printed fashion satires, both of which rely on detailed observation of current dress and manners, afford significant insights into social attitudes at the time of their creation and promoted a growing self-scrutiny among their 'audience'. Today, fashion plates and fashion satires satisfy our desire to know what the past looked like. They are repositories of social and sartorial detail – innovative art forms with their own rich vocabularies. They are also, as Baudelaire noted, an art form fundamentally concerned with the topical, the present moment. Together they can be studied as representations that played an active role, not just in recording fashionable society, but in determining how their readers imagined themselves and understood the world around them.

Style and Satire: Comparing Fashion Plates and Fashion Satires

Studying the fashion satire and fashion plate side by side reveals that the two forms share more than subject matter. Their close correspondence extends to production and distribution: for much of the eighteenth and nineteenth centuries the two genres were products of the same print market, often executed by the same designers and printmakers, issued by the same publishers, and consumed by a shared audience. The eighteenth-century French print merchants, Jacques Esnaut and Michel Rapilly (*fl.*1770–1804), for example, published both fashion plates and fashion satires, as would Parisian publisher Pierre de La Mésangère (1759–1831) in the opening decades of the nineteenth century.

Up until the 1820s, etching – an intaglio printmaking technique, whereby acid-bitten lines on a metal plate are inked to transfer a design to paper – was the primary process used to produce both fashion plates and fashion satires, although different qualities inherent to the technique were exploited according to each artist's purpose. In etching, the artist draws a needle through a soft coating on a printing plate to expose the metal where acid needs to act. This technique affords a more spontaneous and delicate line than the related technique of engraving, in which a burin is used to scoop slivers of

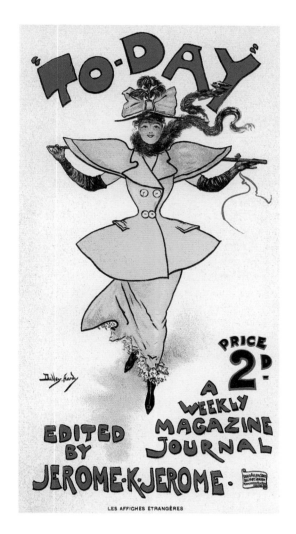

Dudley Hardy (1867–1922)
'To-Day', poster for *To-Day* magazine, London, 1893

Colour lithograph, 190.5 × 297.2 cm
Mary Evans Picture Library

9

metal directly out of the plate. The elegance of many of these fashion plates results from the printmaker's refined use of the etching needle. Satirists such as James Gillray (1756–1815), however, made use of the raw, expressive possibilities of line created when an etching needle scores through the etching ground to animate their compositions. Colour contributed greatly to the visual appeal of both genres, and was crucial to the readers' understanding of the designs being described in fashion plates. Until the 1850s, however, there was no commercially viable process for mass colour printing, and each etched fashion plate or satire was individually coloured by hand, with uncoloured versions also available at a lower price.

From the late eighteenth century through to the 1830s there was a flourishing trade in satirical prints published as relatively large, single sheets. These were sold mainly through print shops catering to a wealthy clientele, although the widespread practice of displaying them in the windows of these shops meant that they also served as a form of street entertainment. Fashion plates, meanwhile, were disseminated first as individual prints and then generally, though not exclusively, as supplementary sheets bound into fashion journals. These were sold directly to the fashionable upper classes, and were also picked up by dressmakers and tailors wishing to inspire their customers. It was the expansion of the periodical press in the mid-nineteenth century, and the development of new commercial printing techniques, that carried both fashion journalism and graphic humour to wider, middle-class audiences. From this period on, graphic satire was integrated within the pages of magazines and journals.

Of the artists and printmakers featured in this book, many shifted seamlessly between the two genres. Artists across the whole period discussed here – from Horace Vernet (1789–1863), who designed fashion plates for publisher Pierre de La Mésangère's long-running, Paris-based fashion magazine the *Journal des dames et des modes* (1797–1839)

and for the *Almanach des modes* (1814–22); to George Barbier (1882–1932), whose opulent fashion plates typify the graphic arts of the Art Deco – also produced prints satirizing the lives and times of their contemporaries. The two genres frequently borrowed from each other. Satirists copied figures directly from fashion plates, and fashion plate illustrators, in turn, looked to the composition of social satires in order to introduce a sense of 'lifestyle' into their plates. The boundaries between the two were often indistinct: when de La Mésangère published Vernet's *Incroyables et Merveilleuses* (1810–18, pp.4, 53) – a deluxe series of hand-coloured plates gently parodying the progressive ensembles of fashionable Paris types – it was not always clear, particularly to subsequent audiences, to which genre the prints belonged. The degree of detail lavished on the realization of the dress itself recalls their designer's alternate role producing straight fashion plates for the *Journal des dames et des modes*.

Fashion plates and fashion satires continued to develop alongside each other over a period of 150 years, sharing the same social, economic and technological environment, and were often in a direct, and highly self-conscious, dialogue with each other. Satirists sometimes attacked, not so much fashion itself, as the way it was presented in fashion plates. Matthew Darly's (*fl.*1750–78) satires of women's coiffures in the print series *Darly's Comic Prints of Characters, Caricatures, Macaronies etc.* (1777, p.35) mimic the format and titles of French printed designs for hairstyles, such as those found in the luxury publication *La Gallerie des modes et costumes français* (1778–87, p.34), which were modelled on those worn by courtiers and the nobility. To English readers, largely unfamiliar with the realities of French court dress, the plates in the *Gallerie des modes* must have seemed almost flights of fancy, and it is this faithful, earnest documentation of even the most outlandish styles that activates Darly's satire – in some cases only a little exaggeration was necessary to make caricatures out of the original fashion plates.

Similarly, at the end of our period, in the mid-1920s, Ettore Tito (1859–1941) gently spoofed the already highly-stylized Art Deco fashion plates of his time (p.75).

Sometimes, fashion plates 'answered back': several fashion satires by James Gillray aped the conventions of fashion plates, of the kind found in British magazine *La Belle Assemblée* (1806–68), and, on at least one occasion, the magazine seems to have acknowledged his satires. In May 1810, Gillray's satirical print, 'The Graces in a high Wind – a Scene taken from Nature, in Kensington Gardens' (pp.50–1), shows three women with their diaphanous gowns blown between their legs and clinging to their buxom bottoms. The issue of *La Belle Assemblée* published a month later remarked on 'the cold easterly winds during the last month', and observed that 'our climate is a terrible enemy to that airy elegant style of dress so well adapted to the light nymph-like figure of our fair country women' – a wry comment that sounds very like a direct nod to Gillray's print.[6]

It made sense for satirists to copy directly from fashion plates in order to create humorous, fashionable figures, their accuracy ensuring that readers would recognize these figures as being absolutely of the moment. One of the female figures in George Cruikshank's (1792–1878) 'Monstrosities of 1822' (published in October of that year, pp.56–7), for example, wears a walking outfit almost identical to that which appeared in the September 1822 issue of *La Belle Assemblée* (p.55).

Fashion plates, in turn, borrowed visual devices from the satirists. The format and topographical setting of tailor Benjamin Read's (*fl.*1820s–40s) large-scale fashion plates, which he began to publish in the mid-1820s, were almost certainly directly inspired by George Cruikshanks annual 'Monstrosities' satires, which mocked the fashions of the preceding year. Cruikshank always set the 'Monstrosities' prints in Hyde Park or nearby, as this was where the fashionable crowd of nineteenth-century London went to see and to be seen, and therefore provided a logic for a plate showing figures grouped together. Read recognized that this principle worked equally well for 'straight' fashion plates and even employed George Cruikshank's brother Robert (1789–1856), also a satirical artist, to draw his plates. The Cruikshanks repaid the compliment – the 'Monstrosities' print of 1827 was lettered as being drawn, 'from Mr B. Read's fashions'.[7]

Often an attack can constitute a form of affirmation. Fashion satire can generalize the experience of the politician who is pleased to be caricatured because it means that he or she is relevant. Indeed, social satires of this period often originated from within the fashionable circles they mocked – it was common practice for aristocratic amateurs to sketch an idea and pass it to an artist such as Gillray, to be worked up.

The Origins and Development of Fashion Plates and Fashion Satire

Although the tradition of graphic satire in Europe dates back to sixteenth-century Italy, fashion satires and the larger body of social satire to which they belong did not emerge in earnest until the eighteenth century, when artists fully grasped the rich potential of dress as a comic device. Previously, few graphic satires dealt with fashion in any systematic way. It was therefore not until the eighteenth century, a period that also witnessed the accelerated growth and diversification of the wardrobe, alongside the increasing commercial development of the fashion industry, that fashion satires came to be produced in great numbers and caricaturists seized on the excesses of, particularly, French fashions, which were adopted throughout the continent and across the Channel. This attention further intensified in the second half of the century – arguably as a direct response to the birth of fashion journalism proper in Britain and France.

The founding of various fashion magazines, a new literary genre devoted to the discussion of fashion and its accoutrements, combined with the sudden influx of unprecedented numbers of fashion-centred images – distributed either in these new journals, or published and sold unbound – brought fashion to the forefront of popular culture as never before and provided a visual framework within which to contemplate, compare and criticize its trappings.[8]

While satirists who addressed this flow of sartorial imagery intended principally to entertain and amuse, there is a moral undercurrent to much of their work. After all, as dress historian Aileen Ribeiro has observed, 'Dress, as an art so closely linked to the body, so revelatory of conscious or unconscious sexuality, is constantly liable to hostile interpretation.'[9]

In Britain, fashion satires were devoured by an appreciative and, for the most part, educated public, whose taste and tolerance for a ribald, incisive humour had been cultivated for decades.[10] This, what is commonly referred to as the 'Golden Age' of graphic satire, saw the rise of artists now synonymous with the genre: William Hogarth (1697–1764); Robert Dighton (1752–1814); James Gillray; Thomas Rowlandson (c.1756–1827); Mary and Matthew Darly (fl.1756–77; fl.1750–78); George Cruikshank; and, later, William Heath (1795–1840). In ancien régime France, however, the press operated under far stricter controls, and the prevailing censorship measures, which dated back to the reign of Louis XIV (1638–1715), did not begin to ease until the revolution in 1789.[11] While fashion caricatures, often targeting the perceived excesses of courtiers and therefore executed under the cover of anonymity, were produced before this period, it was not with the profusion of those seen in Britain. Prints such as 'Promenade de la gallerie du Palais Royal' (The Palais Royal – gallery's Walk, 1787), by Philibert-Louis Debucourt (1755–1832), and Louis Le Coeur's (fl.1784–1825) 'Promenade du

Jardin du Palais Royal' (The Palais Royal Garden Walk, 1787) are celebrated now as examples of pre-revolutionary satire of an altogether more subtle and cautious strain than that practised in Britain. Printed board games that took fashion as their theme, such as publisher Jean Baptiste Crépy's (fl.1753–90) *Le Nouveau Jeu du costume et des coeffures des dames* (New Game of Ladies' Costume and Hairstyles, 1778) offered a mild form of satire – penalizing players who landed on squares illustrating the most extreme fashions.[12] Only in the opening decades of the nineteenth century did French satirists begin to give full vent to their creative powers, as seen in the series of prints *Le Suprême Bon-Ton* (c.1800–02; 1814–16) and *Le Bon Genre* (1801–17, opposite).

If England led the way in humour, then France was the undisputed leader in matters of fashion and taste. It was also a major centre for printmaking and book illustration – even Hogarth insisted on employing French engravers – making it the natural birthplace for fashion journalism in the eighteenth century.[13] Most historians argue that the fashion plate evolved from costume books and plates – illustrative documents of foreign and regional dress, or visual compendiums of curiosities from other lands, the earliest of which dates from 1486: Bernhard von Breydenbach's (1440–97) *Peregrinatio in Terram Sanctam* – which became popular throughout Europe in the sixteenth century.[14] From these developed individually issued plates and *portraits en mode* – portraits of the nobility or celebrated thespians and opera singers, in which dress is made the focus – which began to appear in Paris in the mid- to late seventeenth century. There was no real equivalent in contemporary English print production.[15] Such plates, often coloured after their acquisition, were published in the important French gazette the *Mercure galant* (1672–1724), its successor the *Mercure de France* (1724–1825), and in assorted almanacs and as individual suites of prints.[16] They can be seen as a direct precursor to the true fashion plate – which went beyond a mere record of contemporary

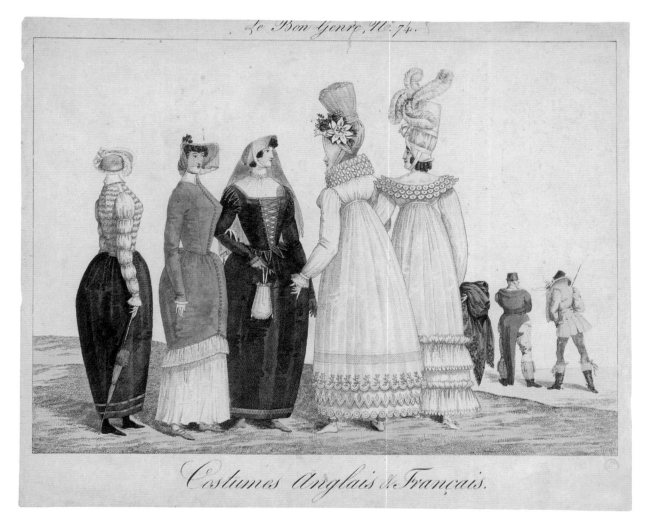

Unknown artist
'[no. 74] Costumes Anglais et Français.' (English and French Dress.),
from the series *Le Bon Genre*, published by Pierre de La Mésangère
(1759–1831), Paris, 1814

Hand-coloured etching, 22 × 26.5 cm. V&A: 23700:1.

dress and was distinguished by its desire 'to guide ladies in
their choice of dress' – as can the range of prints produced
by prominent artists that strayed into depictions of
fashionable attire, often classified as 'costume plates':
works by Wenceslaus Hollar (1607–77), Daniel Rabel
(1578–1637); Jacques Callot (1592–1635); Abraham Bosse
(1604–76); Jean-Antoine Watteau (1684–1721); and Hubert
Gravelot (1699–1773).[17]

The pace of production quickened in the eighteenth century
– the number of fashion-related plates issued in Paris,
for example, grew from a modest figure of 102 between
1600 and 1649, to 1,275 between 1750 and 1799.[18] Jean-
Michel Moreau 'le jeune's' (1741–1814) and Sigmund
Freudenberger's (1745–1801) illustrations for the *Monument
du costume physique et morale*, published in three series
between 1775 and 1783, and ostensibly a *précis* of late-
eighteenth-century society and its dress, were enormously
popular in France and England, and their genre-scene-like
arrangement of fashionable figures pursuing decorative
activities (right) were an early template for the staged
fashion plates that would follow.

From around 1760 onwards, English ladies' pocketbooks
– condensed, portable hybrids of almanac and journal,
designed to be carried about one's person – began including
one or two small, uncoloured fashion plates. As the books
were published in advance of the coming year, these
illustrated fashions of the year that had been.[19] The launches
of various fashion-dedicated periodicals were also attempted
and failed in Paris, in 1728, 1758 and 1768.[20] It is the
founding in London of *The Lady's Magazine* (1770–1837),
the first women's magazine to include fashion plates
(sometimes erroneously referred to as 'The Ladies Magazine',
due to the fact that the fashion plates themselves were
lettered with this title), that is hailed by historians as a
pivotal stage in the continued development of the genre.
In truth, however, its plates were at first not so very
dissimilar to those already found in pocketbooks – that is

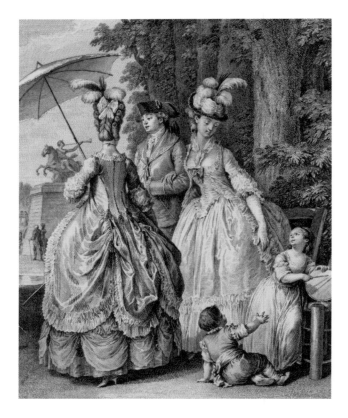

Carl Güttenberg (1743–90), after Jean-Michel Moreau 'le jeune' (1741–1814)
'Le Rendez-vous pour Marly' (The Assignation at Marly), from the
second suite of prints illustrating Nicolas Edme Restif de la Bretonne,
Monument du costume physique et morale de la fin du dix-huitième siècle,
Paris, 1777 (detail)

Etching, 58.8 × 43.8 cm
V&A: E.471–1972. Given by Elizabeth Ison and Anne Gregson in memory
of their uncle, Captain H.R. King.

to say, sparse in number, small, of a mediocre execution and uncoloured. Only towards the end of the century, in around 1790, did the magazine's largely literary content assume a more fashion-dedicated focus, and its plates receive a bright, if somewhat haphazard, wash of colour.

It was not until the founding in Paris some years later of *La Gallerie des modes et costumes français* (1778–87) and *Le Cabinet des modes* (1785–6) that these plates began to resemble what are classically termed 'fashion plates'.[21] These were luxury publications that followed fashions in Paris and at the French court very closely (*La Gallerie des modes* even produced a series of portraits of the royal family) and offered the consumer a choice of either uncoloured plates, or (the more expensive option) delicate, hand-coloured images. The early plates of the short-lived *La Gallerie des modes* in particular, whose publishers boasted of their talented artists, were well drawn and imaginatively composed. Unusually for the fashion plate genre, they also contained a number of provocative plates, perhaps betraying their mixed-sex readership (fashion plates for both sexes were included); the sexually suggestive poses of some of the female figures, the glimpses of bare flesh and perilously low necklines, did not scandalize the French, who had a developed taste for eroticized prints, but would have appeared shockingly risqué to English eyes.

Perhaps the most important development for the fashion plate in the eighteenth century, after the introduction of hand-colouring, was the appearance of serialized publications, allowing trends to be charted on a monthly, or more frequent, basis. The inaugural issue of *Le Cabinet des modes*, for example, expressly laid out the details of its distribution and composition: there were to be 24 issues a year, published at 15-day intervals, each issue comprised of eight pages of text and three etched fashion plates. The reader was, therefore, now apprised of *fortnightly* developments in fashionable dress, with the assistance of visual aids, where before they had expected to receive

updates on a seasonal or yearly basis at best. This regular progression imposed a more rigid, and consistent, schedule on the consumption of fashion, automatically marking trends with a clearly defined lifespan, and inadvertently accelerating the overall cycle of their adoption and disposal. In this way, the commercial interests of the publishers, whose serialized fashion journals were, after all, conceived to encourage a faithful readership and thus turn a greater profit, also dictated the pace of fashion itself.

The new, high-quality, coloured fashion plates often came at a steep price. A subscriber to *Le Cabinet des modes* paid 21 *livres* per annum – no mean sum – placing the publication well beyond the reach of the literate lower-middle classes and rendering it primarily the preserve of the wealthy and leisured. The content was prepared by both male and female journalists, the latter a new phenomenon. Additionally, unlike most of the fashion periodicals that were to follow in the nineteenth century, *Le Cabinet des modes* contained fashion plates and articles aimed at both sexes.[22] Fashions were 'described in a clear and precise manner', and the magazine aimed to give 'an exact and timely knowledge' of both new garments and accessories, while also offering advice on a wide range of other luxury goods: furnishings, interiors, carriages, jewellery, metalwork, and 'generally everything of which fashion offers that is singular, pleasant or interesting'.[23] The presence of plates containing designs for said luxury goods underscores the cultivated readership the publishers sought. The content of its articles, meanwhile, competed with that of more learned journals.[24]

These early fashion periodicals, with their weighty intellectual aspirations, have little in common with the fashion magazines of today; indeed they have no direct modern equivalent. In England, Rudolph Ackermann's *Repository of Arts* (1809–29) declared itself a 'Repository of Arts, Literature, Commerce, Manufactures, Fashions and Politics'. Its January issue in 1814 contained a biography of Mozart; a description of the Pantheon with illustrative plates; an analysis of Napoleonic politics; designs for 'fashionable furniture' in the Empire style; needlework patterns; poetry; reports on the London markets; a meteorological journal; and, finally, fashion plates illustrating ladies' morning and promenade dresses. Similarly, an 1806 issue of British magazine *La Belle Assemblée* – the enormously successful creation of publisher John Bell, which addressed itself 'particularly to the Ladies' – included sections on fine arts, politics, poetry and music; 'biographic sketches of illustrious ladies' (in this issue, Queen Charlotte); needlework patterns; and meditative essays in the form of letters to the editor (including one ominously titled 'Usefulness of an Old Woman').[25] In Germany, Friedrich Justin Bertuch's *Journal des Luxus und der Moden* (1786–1827), followed a similarly literary format.

Among the other influential and lavishly produced periodicals founded during this period was London-based Nikolaus Wilhelm von Heideloff's *Gallery of Fashion* (1790–1822), now synonymous with late Georgian and Regency fashion, which exalted the 'superior elegance of English taste', picturing contemporary dress as it was worn by ladies who 'appear at the routs, the opera, the play-houses, and the concert-rooms; as well as those elegant morning dresses of Hyde Park, and Kensington Gardens.' Heideloff's journal was by far the pinnacle of fashion plate production – without peer on either side of the Channel – and its illustrious subscribers included Queen Charlotte and other members of the British royal family. The plates were issued loose and were of a generous large format, ideally suited for framing and display. Elegant compositions with subtle areas of line and tone were exquisitely realized through etching and aquatint, all beautifully finished by hand with delicate washes of watercolour and gold paint highlights. The plates, which included glimpses of country piles and iconic urban landmarks such as St Paul's Cathedral, London, or evoked fashionable destinations like seaside and spa towns,

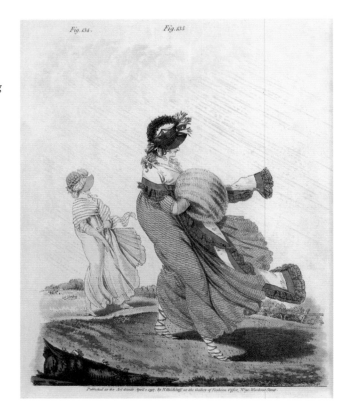

Nikolaus Wilhelm von Heideloff (1761–1837)
'Hyde Park. Morning Dresses', published in the *Gallery of Fashion*, London, 1 April 1797

Hand-coloured etching and aquatint, 29 × 22.5 cm
National Art Library: RC.R.14

16

were of such an exacting, idiosyncratic nature as to include faithful representations of the inclement English weather (opposite).[26]

Such plates, when combined with other highbrow content, reveal publishers' attempts to elevate the status of the fashion journal. Established and well-respected artists were employed to produce fashion plates, which looked to contemporary portraiture, and even history painting, for their cues. The addition of classical vases and statues; the use of lofty settings, including manicured grounds and parks, country houses, even sites of antiquity from the grand tour; and the painterly framing of these compositions, all make palpable allusion to illustrious artistic antecedents while also reflecting something of their viewers' *milieu* (or that to which they aspired). It could also be argued, however, that the increased awareness of fashion that arose from the emergence of fashion plates, and the way in which they groomed their audience to scrutinize dress and its accoutrements – as part of a luxurious and aspirational lifestyle – contributed to the conspicuous use of fashion and accessories to convey the character and status of sitters in portraiture from this period.

Trade and Consumption: The Commercial Contexts of Fashion Plates and Graphic Satires

Fashion plates and periodicals in the eighteenth and early nineteenth centuries provided support and exposure for the luxury trades and, later, the couture industry. They gave specific details about the textiles and accessories depicted (though, traditionally, they were not intended as guides to real wares, so much as observations of garments worn among the fashionable classes), the better to inform a fashionable consumer. The social activities of shopping and promenading had grown in popularity in the eighteenth century, the goal being to display and validate one's fashion sense by disporting oneself before one's peers, and fashion

plates both benefited from and encouraged this culture of spectatorship and consumerism. The portraitist Elisabeth-Louise Vigée Le Brun (1755–1842) would recall, of the streets of pre-revolutionary Paris:

> The side paths were full of immense throngs of pedestrians, enjoying the pastime of admiring or criticizing all the lovely ladies, dressed in their best, who passed in their fine carriages.[27]

Later in the nineteenth century, plates were often lettered with the names and addresses of couturiers and fashion houses, or with small advertisements for other purveyors of fashionable goods. Many fashion journals gained sponsorship or subsidy from fashion houses, and it is therefore unsurprising to find fashion plates with shop interiors as their setting and figures shown browsing or purchasing the wares on offer.[28]

The commercial world also furnished satirists with an important, and subversive, marketplace and social arena: the printseller's shop. Throughout the eighteenth century and the first decades of the nineteenth, this was where one would come to view and purchase both caricatures and fashion plates, and contemporary artists depict the space as a locus of immense, rollicking activity.[29] The shops' expansive windows afforded free entertainment – a motley assembly of people from all classes could gather and discuss the works on display.[30] Here, fashion plate and satire collided and fashionable consumers would find themselves confronted with either their paradigm or their nemesis. In both cases, the fashionable lady or gentleman might enjoy the narcissistic pleasure of seeing him- or herself reflected in the print shop window (overleaf).

Both genres, indeed all classes of print, were plagued by piracy. Fashion plates in particular were copied freely – their elements appropriated and re-assembled – and all with the greatest impunity, for copyright laws were

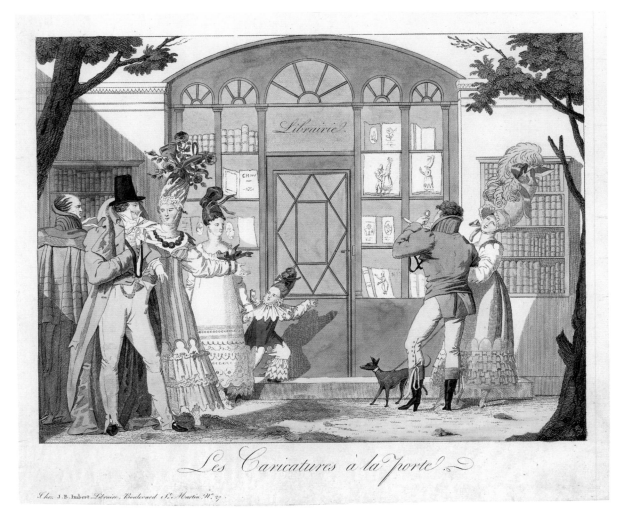

Les Caricatures à la porte.

Unknown artist
'Les Caricatures à la porte.' (Caricatures at the door.),
published by J. B. Imbert (*fl.*1814), Paris, 1814

Hand-coloured etching, 26.5 × 32 cm
Bibliothèque nationale de France, Cabinet des Estampes

still in their infancy in the eighteenth century. Publishers themselves often sold on or exported their printing plates, to be used by others in the trade, among new readers.[31] Such activities being commonplace, viewers today should exercise caution when attempting to read these prints as an exact and faithful record of the fashions they purport to depict; a fashion plate drawn in France, representing the very latest Parisian fashions, could resurface in a German publication some weeks later, with new lettering identifying it as an example of fashionable dress from Italy.[32] This practice continued into the nineteenth century, although it was principally fashion plates originating in France that were copied or reissued – they were often detached from their original descriptions in the process.

Fashion plates were as much a promotional tool for the printing industry as they were for garments. They helped to sell magazines by providing constant updates on a subject that was of interest to an elite readership. Pages filled with the most up-to-date dress (whether as part of actual fashion news, or scenes and satires of social life) were one of the most effective means publishers had of making their magazines feel of the moment. Fashion, meanwhile, by appearing in print, was tracked to the commercial rhythms of the periodical market. An image was turned into an event by the very fact of publication – it appeared on a particular day and existed in multiple copies that were viewed separately, but simultaneously, by many people. The temporality of the fashion plate was important: plates nearly always had the month inscribed at the bottom and periodicals often repeated the date of issue on every page.

Their topicality aside, fashion plates were desirable and luxurious objects in their own right. Exquisite printing, careful hand-colouring and high-quality paper meant that, in the eighteenth century especially, they were collected and displayed as decorative objects. Gillray's satirical series, *Progress of the Toilet* (1810, right), though conceived

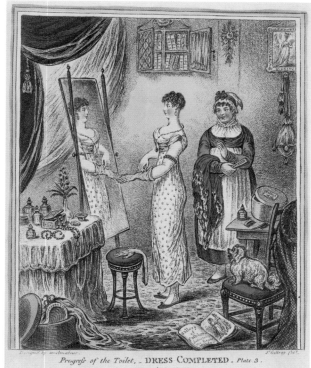

James Gillray (1756–1815)
'Progress of the Toilet. – Dress Completed. Plate 3.',
published by Hannah Humphrey (*c*.1745–1818), London, 1810

Hand-coloured etching, 30.7 × 24.2 cm
V&A: 1232(84)–1882. Jones Bequest.

19

for humorous ends, nonetheless gives us some idea of how fashion plates were used by their readers. In the third print in the series, the reader spies a framed fashion plate mounted on the wall of a fashionable young woman's dressing room, while another, presumably more current, plate is still bound into a journal that lies open on the floor, having played its role in the 'progress of the toilet'. There is a sense in this print that, framed in her mirror, the woman has herself become a fashion plate. The punchline, of course, is that, by effecting this transformation, she has also made herself into an object of satire.

A plate from an album compiled by Barbara Johnson (1738–1925) in the eighteenth century, a unique survival (right), gives us further valuable information as to how fashion plates were consumed in this period. Plates drawn predominantly from ladies' pocketbooks have been pasted into the album, alongside various silk samples, with dates and detailed annotations. Their size made pocketbook fashion plates highly collectable: Sarah Sophia Banks (1744–1818), sister to English scientist Sir Joseph Banks (1743/4–1820), assembled over 400 in her collection of prints and ephemera.[33]

Fashion plates did not include the technical information required to actually make the garments depicted, which would usually have required the skilled interpretation of a professional dressmaker or tailor. Nevertheless, by addressing the customer's desire directly, fashion plates affected people's relationship with their dressmaker or tailor, influencing how they made their choices and communicated their wishes. More fashion plates were printed for women's fashions than for men's – a reflection of the fact that a greater volume of magazine titles dealing with fashion were addressed specifically to women (although that is not to say that men didn't read them). There were monthly fashion magazines for men, such as *The Gentleman's Magazine of Fashion* (1828–94). However, many fashion plates dealing with men's fashions were marketed to tailors, along with

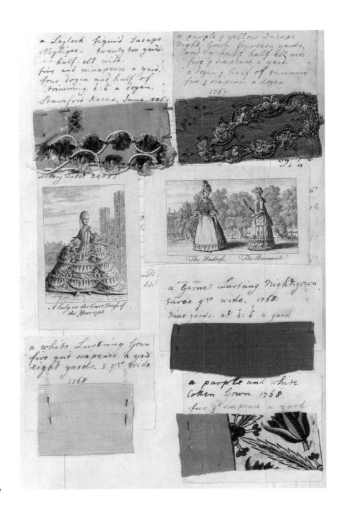

Page from an album of textile samples and fashion plates compiled by Barbara Johnson (1738–1825) between 1746 and 1823, England, 1767–8

Etchings and fragments of woven silks and printed cotton, 38.1 × 24.7 cm
V&A: T.219–1973

patterns and cutting information – a model that would migrate to women's publishing as the nineteenth century wore on.

Fashion Lessons: Social Etiquette and Anxiety

Fashion journals and manuals in book form promoted correct social conduct alongside fashionable wares, schooling the reader, not just in fashionable dress, but in social mores. Their instructive tone often reflected other, more established, didactic literature (usually directed at women): etiquette guides; scientific, religious and social treatises on marriage and family; and moralizing biographies and novels centred on prominent women of 'good character'.[34] But above all, fashion plates, with their lengthily-lettered titles and comprehensive explanatory texts, were conceived as a guide to a sartorial and social world that was becoming increasingly elaborate, even bewildering, in its complexity.[35]

Over the course of the eighteenth century, people of all classes came to own more articles of clothing than ever before, prompting society hostess Lady Frances Anne Crewe (1748–1818) to observe to a friend in 1785, 'What a puzzling matter Dress is become within these two or three years.'[36] This was an age, however enlightened, in which dress continued to be governed by a strict etiquette; it was not necessarily that one enjoyed following fashions, as that it was a social obligation.[37] Auguste Caron's manual on female dress and beauty, the *Toilette des dames* (1806), translated and published in London by W.H. Wyatt in 1808, expounded:

> The love of dress is in itself a laudable propensity. It indicates in women, and likewise in men, a love of order and propriety, esteem for themselves, and respect for others. People who have profoundly studied the world have even remarked that there is an invariable coincidence between the character and the dress of a person.[38]

Conversely, the tyrannical grip of fashion and wanton extravagance, Caron argued, were to be censured: 'Fashion and luxury! These are the bane of good taste, of private happiness, and public morals.'[39] People of fashion walked a fine line between fashionable, correct dress and that of, in our modern idiom, the 'fashion victim'.

As the means to travel and witness changing fashions for oneself extended only to a privileged few, fashion plates and magazines were all the more pertinent to those residing far from city centres. A prescriptive and detailed guide was necessary if the woman or man of fashion were to successfully avoid the many perils and pitfalls of the fashionable body, and relay their sartorial requirements with absolute precision to their dressmakers, tailors, perruquiers and milliners. Fashion plates, easily reproduced and disseminated, played a part in accelerating both the adoption and relentless renewal of fashions, and contemporaries registered their growing concern with the chaotic pace of the new culture of fashion. In her 1796 novel *Camilla*, Frances Burney (1752–1840) wrote: 'no contagion spreads with greater certainty nor greater speed than that of fashion; slander itself is not more sure of promulgation.'[40] Along with this concern about the speed of change came the constant anxiety of hovering between the fashionable and the passé: 'As good be out of the world as out of the fashion,' Lord Chesterfield opined.[41] It is the notion that fashion might be inherently arbitrary, even absurd, that is underlined by satires such as 'In Fashion. Out of Fashion.' (overleaf), where the reader is invited to compare a 'fashionable' woman, whose silhouette is grossly exaggerated by her attire and accessories, unfavourably with her 'unfashionable' (but, it is suggested, more sincere and honest) counterpart: a young country girl.

The high artifice of fashion plates provoked an overwhelming and cautionary response from satirists. A particular target for scorn was the 'macaroni' – a term first used in London in 1764 to describe an aristocratic English man who adopted the affected fashions, coiffures and

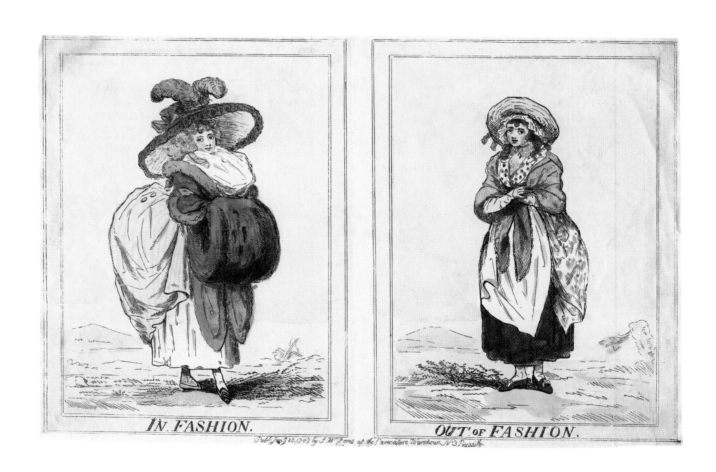

IN FASHION.   OUT OF FASHION.

Pub.d Jan.y 13.1787 by S.W. Fores at the Caricature Warehouse N.o 3 Piccadilly.

Unknown artist
'In Fashion. Out of Fashion.', published by S.W. Fores (1761–1838),
London, 7 January 1787

Hand-coloured etching, 27 × 41.2 cm
The Lewis Walpole Library

deportment of his Italian and French contemporaries – usually as prompted by experiences on the grand tour. Over the years, its meaning expanded to denote a general extravagance and excess in dress bordering on absurdity.[42] The figure of the macaroni became a trope popularly used by satirists to signal vanity and elitism, playing to contemporary moralists' argument that fashion posed a genuine threat to public ethics and common sense.

Over the decades, other stock figures of fun would join the macaroni, including the fop, the dandy and the female macaroni, who inconveniences her partner with patently ridiculous attire – notably paniers and towering coiffures. The country girl or boy transformed, or corrupted, was another popular stereotype. 'Heyday! Is this my daughter Anne' (1779), and its pendant 'Is this my son Tom' (1774), by Francis Adams, and 'The Farmer's Daughter's Return from London' (1777), are typical of satires showing the children of 'honest' country folk rendered unrecognizable to their horrified parents after yielding to the 'vanities' of the city. Other prints emphasized the growing divide between the dress of the current generation and the more modest, sober attire of their grandparents – as demonstrated by Rushworth's 'My Grandmother peeping out of her Grave' (1786). Satirists also disdained those who dressed outside their immediate age group or, worse, those who dressed above their social station, posing an alarming threat to the social status quo; examples include Thomas Rowlandson's 'An Old Ewe Drest Lamb Fashion' (1810) and Darly's 'A speedy & Effectual preparation for the next world' (1777). A letter from a concerned reader to the editor of *The Gentleman's Magazine and Historical Chronicle* (1736–1833) in 1801 grumbled of the daughters of yeoman families:

> Instead of dishing butter, feeding poultry, or curing bacon, the avocations of these young ladies at home are, studying dress, attitudes, novels, French, and musick, whilst the fine ladies their mothers sit lounging in parlours adorned with the fiddle-faddle fancy-works of their fashionable daughters.[43]

Tradespeople associated with the fashion industry, who arguably encouraged such aspirational behaviour, did not escape the scrutiny of the satirists either, and are treated with a particular contempt; the draper, seamstress, shop girl, milliner and tailor – all were styled as cunning and ruthless adversaries, obsequious yet mercenary, complicit in the charade of fashion and taking every opportunity to swindle the vulnerable consumer.

Another of the most persistent themes in satire over this whole period, and one that endures even today, was that of the French/English divide – the political opposition of the two nations expressed through their diverging approaches to dress and deportment. French satirists portrayed the English as dull-witted, backward simpletons, their features coarse and figures misshapen, while the English saw the French as mincing, posturing, weak-minded fools, their emaciated forms mere vessels for the most conspicuous profligacy. One potential reason for this slander, from the English side at least, was the fashionable set's slavish imitation of French fashions in the face of a broad and deep-seated resentment of French cultural ascendancy. Political controversies also inflected many satires – recent research has shown that the outsized feather headdresses worn by many women of 'The Quality' in London in the 1770s were damned by caricaturists as a fashion imported from France, and likened to the feather headdresses of Native Americans, at a time when unrest was growing in the American colonies.[44]

On a more intimate scale, a theme consistently mined for satire is the relationship between art, fashion and the body. A number of Gillray's satires in the early nineteenth century mocked the classical flavour of women's diaphanous gowns and the corresponding fashion plates, in which artists referenced neoclassical statuary (pp.49, 50–1). Conversely, satirists in the early ninteenth century responded to more restrictive styles of dress and criticized fashionable clothing for destroying the naturally beautiful shape of the body.

In George Cruikshank's satirical print 'Monstrosities of 1822', the classical-style bronze of Achilles by Richard Westmacott standing in Hyde Park, London (inaugurated a few months before Cruikshank's satire was published) serves as a counterpoint to the men promenading around it, whose bodies are moulded into awkward shapes by their constrictive clothing. The presence of the martial statue casts aspersion on their masculinity – while the fashionably clothed body is compared unfavourably with the classical nude, a genre revered as enshrining the ideal proportions of the human figure. An opposition is set up between an absolute, 'natural' ideal of beauty (the province of art), and the ephemeral and artificial aesthetic of modern dress (the province of fashion).

The stiff-corseted silhouettes of women's fashions in the mid-nineteenth century, similarly, lent themselves to this theme. In a drawing published in *Punch* (1841–1992) in 1870, 'The Venus of Milo; or, Girls of Two Different Periods', George Du Maurier (1834–96) showed a group of smartly dressed young women crowded around the Venus de Milo (at this time, considered to be one of the most important works of art in existence), exclaiming in horror over her figure and proportions, as judged against the fashionable silhouette of the day: 'Look at her big foot! Oh, what a waist! – and what a ridiculous little head'. The joke is on the blinkered women, who approach the Venus not as a timeless beauty, but as a contemporary, who does not measure up to the standards of the modern fashionable body. Du Maurier offers women's adherence to fashion as evidence of their lack of capacity for artistic criticism and abstract analysis – presented with a great work of art, all they can think about is fashion.

In the same year, however, the *Englishwoman's Domestic Magazine* (1852–79) – a popular women's title that included fashion plates and fashion news – published an engraving using the same conceit as that in *Punch*, though with the humour weighted differently (right). In this version,

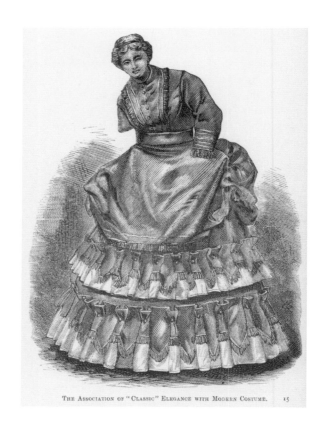

THE ASSOCIATION OF "CLASSIC" ELEGANCE WITH MODERN COSTUME. 15

Unknown illustrator

'The Association of "Classic" Elegance with Modern Costume.' published by the *Englishwoman's Domestic Magazine* in *Figure Training, or, Art the Handmaid of Nature*, London, 1871

Wood engraving, 12 × 18 cm

National Art Library: 24.D.31

the Venus is dressed in a fashionable gown, which, the magazine argues, clearly shows 'how inappropriate and inelegant not to say dowdy even a perfectly-elaborated modern costume would look when worn by a lady of ancient Greece'.[45] In Du Maurier's print, Venus stares down the modern misses. The *Englishwoman's Domestic Magazine*, however, presents her as irrelevant to the modern age. The statue, in this image, distorts the line of the dress and is made to appear hunched and awkward; the fashion and the artwork show each other to be equally artificial ideals. Dressing up the Venus de Milo was a small act of cultural subversion, challenging the idea of there being a natural or authentic body underneath the constructions of civilization.

New Technologies and New Audiences: The Expansion of the Periodical Press in the mid-Nineteenth Century

Throughout the 1820s and 1830s, a wave of new fashion journals emerged. They began to shed their literary pretensions and focus shifted from the affluent reader to the aspirant. The author of the book *The Whole Art of the Dress! Or, the Road to Elegance and Fashion At the Enormous Saving of Thirty Per Cent!!!* (1830), whose guide was pitched at 'the middling orders of society', advised 'For those of our readers, if any such perchance there be, desirous of following the very height of the town, they have only to take in a monthly periodical, entitled *Bell's Gentlemen's Fashions*.'[46]

This was the beginning of a process of democratization in fashion journalism, which accelerated from the mid-century, amid an explosion in periodical publishing – itself brought about by the industrialization of printing processes, the abolition of taxes on paper, and the wider distribution made possible by newly built rail networks. Illustrated newspapers and periodicals, in particular, proliferated in Britain, as the development of wood engraving, a relief-printing technique,

meant that blocks bearing images could be printed alongside moveable metal type in a single operation. A far more economical process than preparing separately etched plates to be bound into a journal, this meant that black-and-white illustrations could be integrated with set type (rather than engraved text) on a single page. In France, the concurrent development of commercial lithographic printing also acted as a stimulus to popular illustration. In lithography an image is held on a printing surface as greasy marks – the lines to be printed do not need to be etched or cut around (as in wood engraving). This makes it a highly versatile technique, capable of reproducing freehand drawing.

The periodical press now reached a wider reading public than ever before. A major consequence was that both fashion journalism and graphic satire were forced to adapt to a new, bourgeois morality – in particular, the new 'cult' of domesticity. British magazine *Punch* developed a new brand of 'amiable humour' that eschewed the passionate and aggressive qualities of humour (such as satire and irony) that had previously characterized graphic satire in Britain, and was proud of its suitability for middle-class drawing rooms. *Punch* led the field of humorous journalism in Britain for the rest of the century and had the most prestigious artists on its staff – many publishers began to imitate its tone. The shift towards 'amiable humour' required not only polite subject matter, but also a style of illustration less vulgar and violent in its lines of its expression. By the 1830s, singly issued satirical prints had disappeared and the acerbic etchings of Gillray, Cruikshank and their contemporaries gave way to mildly humorous social scenes, more or less elegantly drawn by the likes of John Leech (1817–64), John Tenniel (1820–1914) and George Du Maurier.[47] Indeed, graphic satire in Britain arguably lost much of its colour in both the literal and metaphorical senses of the word – the large print runs now being produced meant that hand colouring was not viable and sketches only appeared within periodicals as relatively small, black-and-white engravings.

The format of *Punch* was based on that of French satirical newspaper *Le Charivari* (1832–1937) and *Punch* was subtitled 'The London Charivari'. In 1835, the French government had banned political satire and *Le Charivari* henceforth concentrated on satires of social life, which in turn became more biting. In a reversal of the situation at the turn of the nineteenth century, it was now the expressive and unsentimental satires of French artists such as Charles Vernier (1831–87) and Honoré Daumier (1808–79) that appeared bolder than their British counterparts.

While periodicals were the primary vehicle for graphic satires in the second half of the century, new technologies also presented other outlets for humour. Illustrated music-sheet covers for popular songs composed on all manner of light, topical subjects were printed using colour lithography and would have been displayed on the music stands of household pianos while they were still current. These encompassed fashion themes with humorous mileage, such as the fashion for vast crinoline skirts; or 'bloomerism', referring to 'bloomers', or trousers for women (really divided skirts), which were proposed by dress reformers in the 1850s as a loose and healthy alternative to long skirts (p.60).

Towards the end of the nineteenth century, technological developments in mechanized printing, together with growing demand for innovations in advertising, led to a flood of large-scale colour posters on the streets of wealthy European capitals such as London and Paris. Images of desirable, fashionable women were used to sell all manner of products. In Britain, at the turn of the century, Dudley Hardy (1867–1922) produced a number of such posters, featuring chic and exuberant young women (p.9). His biographer records a telling incident in which Hardy met a 'coster-lass', or fruitseller, decked out in a bright yellow costume, replicating the attire of a woman in one of his poster designs.[48] She had in effect used the poster as a giant and accessible fashion plate. Advertising was

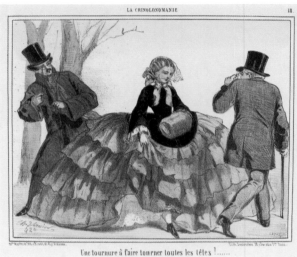

Charles Vernier (1831–87)
'Une tournure à faire tourner toutes les têtes!' (A figure to turn every head!), plate no. 18 from *La Crinolomanie* (Crinolomania), published by *Le Charivari*, Paris, 1856

Hand-coloured lithograph, 20.9 × 25.9 cm
V&A: 23702.A.3

beginning to play an important role in the communication of style and Hardy was typical of a generation of artists whose work spanned not only painting and humorous magazine illustration, but press advertising and poster design.

As the periodical press expanded in the mid-nineteenth century, the genre of the women's magazine continued to develop apace. Many new titles appeared and fashion news was one of the pillars of their content. However, just as *Punch* had domesticated its humour, some repositioning was occasionally required to accommodate fashion content to the middle-class ideal of the 'separate spheres' of the two genders, which defined women's role as domestic. The *Englishwoman's Domestic Magazine*, for example, emphasized active household management as much as appearance. The magazine began selling paper patterns for the actual garments depicted in its fashion plates so that, for the first time, the reader was given all the information needed to replicate them through her own domestic skill. She could imagine herself as both thrifty housekeeper and fashionable lady.[49]

Victorian moralists, however, still accused fashion of being disruptive to domestic bliss and social harmony. An article published in the *Saturday Review* in 1868, 'The Girl of the Period' by Eliza Lynn Linton, raised alarm by suggesting that respectable young women were now modelling their dress on that of courtesans. Linton described this as a corruption of the 'fair young English girl', who used to be 'a tender mother, an industrious housekeeper, a judicious mistress'.[50] 'Imitation of the demi-monde in dress,' she claimed, leads to 'slang, bold talk and general fastness; to the love of pleasure and indifference to duty; to the desire of money before either love or happiness; to uselessness at home...' The ensuing debate spawned a large number of verbal and visual satires, including a whole magazine, *The Girl of the Period Miscellany*, which ran for nine months and was packed with humorous illustrations.

Since periodicals in general now carried a far higher quota of images than previously, fashion plates inevitably appeared alongside a variety of other types of illustration, including social scenes, illustration to poems and serialized fiction and, increasingly, advertisements, many of which were fashion-related – advertisements for corsetières and innovations such as sewing machines and ready-to-wear clothing. Coloured fashion plates, however, where they appeared, remained visually distinct – they continued to be added as separate, hand-coloured sheets, while other illustrations were printed alongside text. They therefore retained their aura of exclusivity and the crucial capacity to communicate the colour of garments and textiles. Although fashion plates were being produced in Britain, plates sourced from France added caché to a magazine and it remained important for British publications to evoke links with Paris, which was re-asserting its claim to be a capital of fashion during the Second Empire thanks to the luxurious court of Napoleon III (1808–73) and the establishment of the influential couturiers House of Worth. Even during the brief, troubled tenure of the socialist Paris Commune, satirists joked that British women were still obtaining their fashionable accessories from Paris via balloon post.[51] The *Englishwoman's Domestic Magazine* obtained its fashion plates from Jules David (1808–92), one of the most prestigious and masterful French illustrators of fashion plates. A surviving design for such a plate, dating from 1866, bears a pencilled inscription containing explicit instructions to the engraver to 'produce a bright plate', with 'a highly finished yet light background', and to take heed that 'all details be precisely rendered' – a testimony to the continued care given to these small works of art.[52]

The composition of fashion plates also became increasingly self-aware in this period. This gave rise to compositions of the type found in the *Journal des demoiselles* (1833–1922), where a modish young woman is shown consulting a fashion plate (overleaf). The plate thus endorses itself as one of the accessories of the fashionable woman, and highlights the way in which fashion plates encouraged their, predominantly female viewers, to adopt a dual position – rehearsing the simultaneous roles of viewer and viewed (compare this with Gillray's satire of the vain miss, p.19). The public settings of eighteenth-century plates – expansive grounds and gardens – gave way in the nineteenth century to more elaborate and aspirational spaces: the museum, the art gallery, the ballroom, concert hall and well-appointed domestic interior. These sites served both to provide the reader with some direction as to which form of dress was appropriate for which occasion – what to wear to the opera or to afternoon tea, for instance – and, by depicting milieux suggesting wealth and privilege, to proffer a comforting, fantasy vision of a quixotic world peopled by immaculately dressed figures.

The periodical press of Victorian England, like the eighteenth-century print shop window before it, was a space where people encountered themselves both in fashion plates and fashion satires. How then would they have made sense of these images that seem to offer aspiration on the one hand and admonition on the other? A fascinating image through which to consider this question is the humorous engraving 'Flirtations in the Authors' Workshop.' (1861, p.30), by the sisters Florence and Adelaide Claxton (*fl.*1840–79), which was published as a stand-alone illustration in *The Queen* (1851–1958), an upmarket womens' newspaper. The growth of the periodical press during this period, it is worth noting, provided an important commercial outlet for female artists. Florence and Adelaide Claxton were two of the first women to draw professionally for magazines and journals in Britain, while, in France, the four Colin sisters were among the most celebrated fashion plate illustrators of their day.[53]

The illustration in question shows two fashionably dressed women in crinolines in the domed Reading Room of the British Museum. The opening of the Reading Room four years previously had greatly increased public access to the Museum's library and included a section for the exclusive

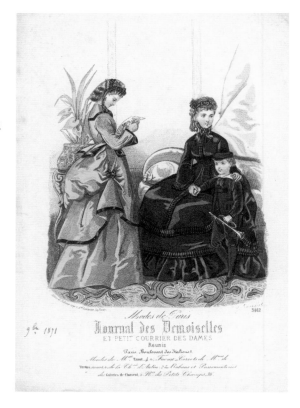

A. Carrache (*fl.*1852–71), after Laure Noël (1827–78)
Untitled, published in the *Journal des demoiselles*, Paris, November 1871

Hand-coloured litho-engraving, 29.2 × 19.2 cm

V&A: E.1353–2011. Given by Mrs Jacqueline Simpson.

use of women. Female presence in the library, however, attracted criticism, as a letter in *The Times* the following year sets out:

> Many of them [women] invade the other portions of the room and mingle with us male students, to our very great discomfort, for they gossip not a little and flirt and ogle a good deal. I do not think, speaking both as a literary man and a 'paterfamilias' that it is a desirable thing that young ladies should frequent the Museum at all as readers.[54]

The Claxton's illustration visualizes just this scenario and foregrounds the women's dresses in a way that would have immediately evoked the ubiquitous crinoline satires of the day, in which women wearing the offending fashion inconvenienced men by taking up too much space. The two women in the Claxtons' illustration reproduce the composition and calm poise of two figures in fashion plates; they are an image of fashion inserted into a scholarly, male, domain and their fashionability marks them out as dilettantes. The illustration could be read, like that letter in *The Times*, as challenging women's right to be in the library at all. But, as an image drawn by women for a female audience, who may well have recognized themselves in it, might it have been interpreted in a different light?

The British Museum Reading Room was one of the new semi-public spaces in London (including shopping arcades, museums and the like) that middle-class women could take advantage of as sites of respectable leisure, and this illustration visualizes them occupying it. The two women depicted have a powerful presence – they fill the centre of the picture and stand while most of the men sit. A much earlier print, by George Cruikshank, shows the British Museum print room, with a group of male connoisseurs (most of them standing) clustered around the centre of a table while a lone woman perches awkwardly in the corner, almost forced out of the image.[55] Although the crinoline was frequently presented by satirists as a symptom of

women's essential vanity and irrationality, in the Claxtons' image the women's expansive skirts equally represent a claim to space and a refusal to be marginalized.

Graphic satire is rarely fixed or stable in its meaning; a satire will be read in divergent ways, and can be rejected or simply ignored. The scholar Julia Thomas has pointed out that condemning a fashion creates the possibility that wearing it becomes a form of resistance. *Punch* led a 10-year-long graphic war against the crinoline, with the magazine promising readers that it would provide a laughing cure for 'crinolineomania'. Its failure to eradicate or stigmatize the trend, however, provides a clear demonstration that satire is never able to actually censor fashion. Rather, the treatment of the crinoline is an example of satire's ability to turn a fashion into a potent cultural symbol by investing it with social and moral anxieties. Crinolines were in fashion at a time when middle-class women were claiming a greater stake in public life – their legal personae, financial and sexual rights and their opportunities for employment were all prominent topics of public debate. Satirical images dealing with these issues intersected with images of women literally (and often disruptively) expanding their sphere.[56]

The End of an Era: The Decline of the Fashion Plate

Continuous innovations in publishing and printing technology meant that the fashion plate as a distinct form had a finite life span. Vyvyan Holland dates the demise of the hand-coloured fashion plate to 1899, after which period they deteriorated immeasurably in quality.[57] This decline can, in part, be ascribed to the advent of photography, which resulted in the substitution of fashion photographs for fashion plates and the development of photomechanical printing techniques. The invention of 'the New Art', by William Henry Fox Talbot (1800–77) in 1835 posed an unprecedented challenge to all the graphic arts. From the 1880s, fashion photography was being used as a resource

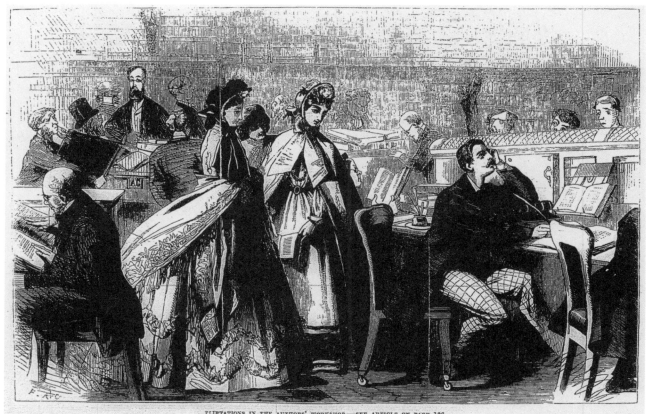

FLIRTATIONS IN THE AUTHORS' WORKSHOP.—SEE ARTICLE ON PAGE 106.

Florence and Adelaide Claxton (*fl.*1840–79)
'Flirtations in the Authors' Workshop.', published in *The Queen*,
London, 1861

Wood engraving, dimensions unknown
British Library Newspaper Archive

by fashion plate engravers, becoming widespread in fashion magazines themselves around 1905, where it was still usually coupled with fashion illustrations.[58]

Photographs provided unparalleled accuracy and detail at a fraction of the cost and labour of fashion plates but, initially at least, sacrificed much of their charm and artistic merit. Publishers responded to this obstacle by styling fashion photographs as if they were fashion plates, leading to images no less contrived or manipulated than their predecessors, as seen in one of the first publications to introduce fashion photography, *Mode Pratique* (1892–1938).[59] Where fashion plates did continue to be used, many were often mere photomechanical copies of prints or illustrations. The French magazine *Les Modes* (1901–37) came to be known for its elegant fashion photography, and designers including Charles Frederick Worth, Jeanne Paquin and Georges Dœuillet began to have their fashions photographed for its pages.[60]

For a brief idyllic interlude in the early twentieth century, however, from about 1912 to 1932, the fashion plate experienced a revival in the lavish publications *Les Choses de Paul Poiret vues par Georges Lepape* (1911), the *Gazette du Bon Ton* and *Art Goût Beauté* (1920–33). George Barbier's designs for these, the *Modes et manieres d'aujourd'hui* (1912–22) and the five jewel-like volumes of *Falbalas & fanfreluches: Almanach des modes présentes, passées et futures* (1922–6), were all realized through *pochoir*, a costly hand-stencilling technique largely responsible for the graphic identity and aesthetic of Art Deco. The *Gazette du Bon Ton* actively departed from the large mechanized print runs of its time and was produced in small, hand-coloured editions.[61] 'André Edouard Marty's (1882–1974) designs for the *Modes et manières d'aujourd'hui* epitomize the sophistication and thoughtfulness of the plates found in these publications. Featured in an issue from 1919, one plate shows an elegant young woman looking out to sea, enjoying the sensation of the wind in her cloak (back cover).

Readers would have identified with the sense of release and rebirth suggested by the image, published as Europe was just emerging from the grip of the First World War. Despite being financed by the couture houses themselves, the cost of producing such luxury fashion journals became untenable and, by 1932, the last had closed its doors forever.[62] Fashion plates continued to appear with some irregularity throughout the 1930s but were finally eclipsed in the 1940s by photography, fashion illustration and fashion advertising.

Graphic fashion satire also receded in both visibility and popularity, as modern audiences' reading patterns changed and, turning away from the satirical journal, they sought humour in the new and more spontaneous media of radio, television and film. In the increasingly liberal and fast-paced twentieth century, dress was no longer the focus of moral comment it had once been and attacks on fashion diminished in frequency and fervour.[63] Various social and economic factors contributed to this shift, effectively neutralizing fashion as a pressing subject of moral concern.

Today, fashion plates and fashion satires remain highly collectable works of art, winning over new audiences with their exacting and entertaining visions of our fashion and social history. Rather than merely idiosyncratic relics of another time, these prints continue to fascinate us because we recognize in them the follies and fancies of our own time, perhaps even more than we would care to admit.

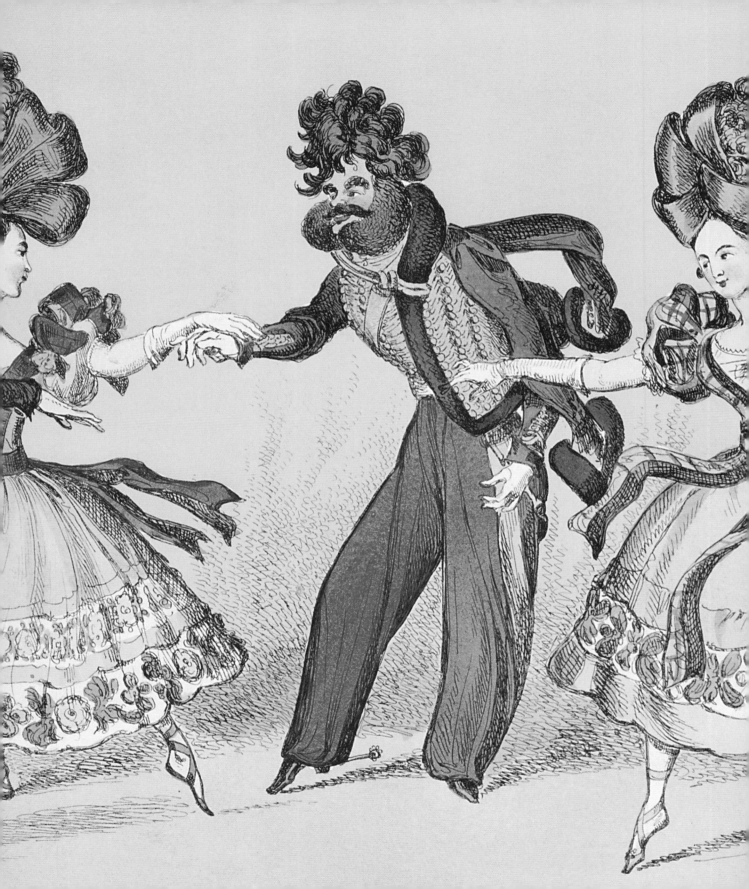

PLATES

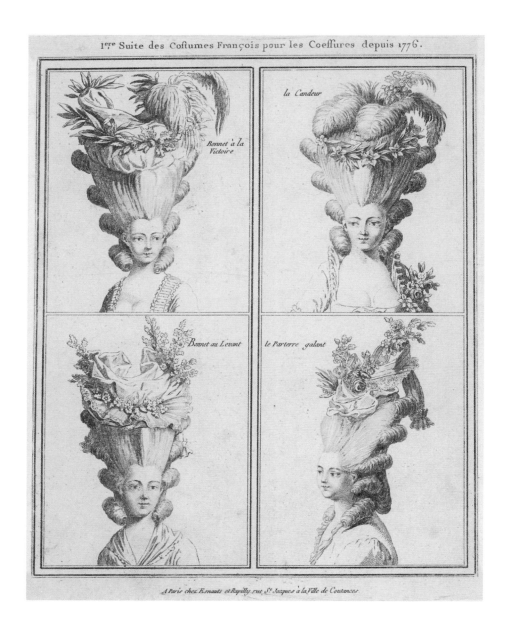

Nicolas Dupin (*fl.*1776–89), after Claude-Louis Desrais (1746–1816)
Untitled, from *1ere Suite des Costumes François pour les Coeffures depuis 1776.* (1st Suite of French styles for Coiffures since 1776.), published in *La Gallerie des modes et costumes français*, Paris, 1778

Etching, 26.4 × 20.3 cm
V&A: 24923.11

Fashionable women in the eighteenth century augmented their own, natural hair by attaching false hairpieces and toupées to a wire structure, or 'cap', which they fastened to the head, adding volume through the use of wool pads, and securing the additions with liberal applications of pomade and powder. For more elaborate concoctions, of the kind pictured here, only a wig would suffice.[1] These were intricately assembled and decked with flowers, ribbons, bows, feathers and jewels. Queen Marie-Antoinette (1755–93) was the most notorious proponent of this fashion.[2]

34

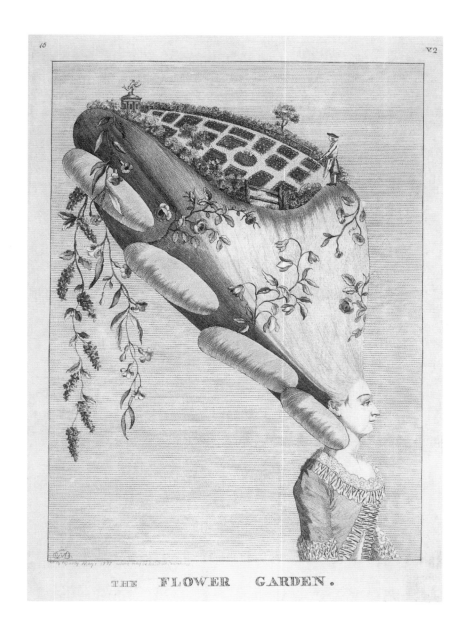

THE FLOWER GARDEN.

Matthew Darly (*fl.*1750–78)
'The Flower Garden.', from the series *Darly's Comic Prints*
of Characters, Caricatures, Macaronies etc., published
by Matthew Darly, London, 1 May 1777

Etching, 35.2 × 24.7 cm
V&A: E.2293–1966

The extreme hairstyles of the 1770s were easy sport for satirists
and more eighteenth-century satirical prints were dedicated to this
particular fashion than almost any other. This coiffure, 'The Flower
Garden', is tended by a miniature gardener and even contains a folly:
a temple to Mercury visible in the distance. This may seem humorous
exaggeration but, in Paris, the duchesse de Lauzun was noted to have
worn a similarly contrived wig, consisting of a landscape in relief,
complete with ducks, a windmill and a miller leading his donkey.[3]

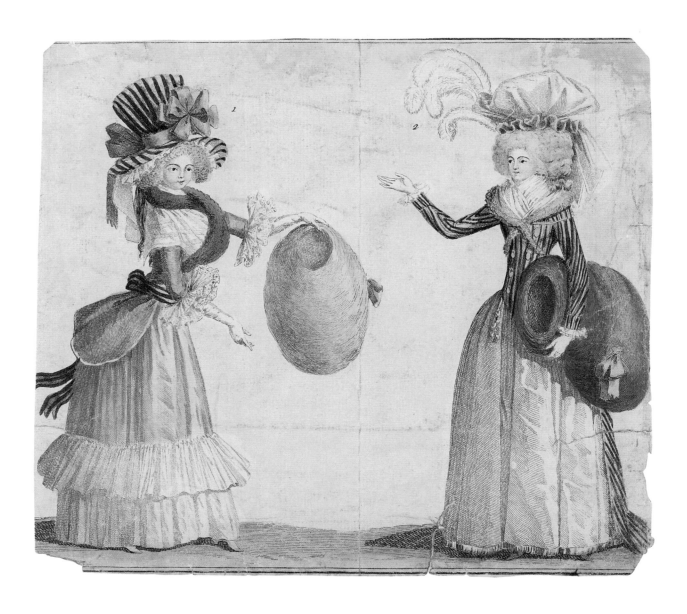

A.B. Duhamel (1736–1800), after Claude-Louis Desrais (1746–1816)
Figs 1 and 2, published in *Le Magasin des modes nouvelles françaises et anglaises*, Paris, December 1787

Hand-coloured etching (fragment), 19 × 10.5 cm
V&A: E.988–1959. Given by Mr. James Laver, CBE.

In the 1780s, excessively large fur muffs were an accessory sported by men and women alike. Fur was necessary in an age without adequate heating, but it could also be decorative – furs were embellished with ribbons or tied about one's person, and were even fragranced. They were made from an extraordinarily broad range of pelts, including bear, fox, mink, otter, sable, skunk and squirrel and, by virtue of their size and expense, became signifiers of fashionability and status.

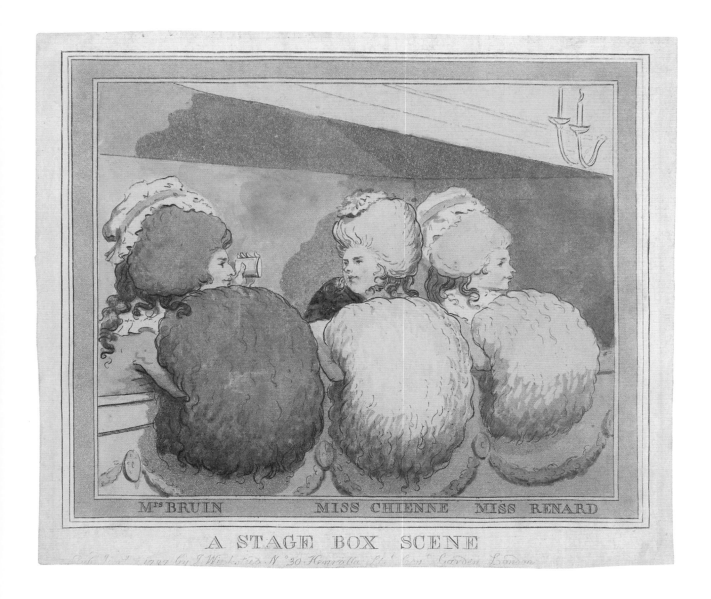

MRS BRUIN   MISS CHIENNE   MISS RENARD

A STAGE BOX SCENE

Unknown artist
'A Stage Box Scene', published by James Wicksteed,
London, 1 January 1787

Hand-coloured etching, 19.5 × 23 cm
V&A: E.3888–1902. Given by Mr. T. Armstrong, C.B.

From their vantage point in a theatre box reserved for ladies, three
fashionable women with oversized fur muffs survey their fellow audience
members, all the while forming an arresting tableau themselves. Their
humorous titles: 'Mrs Bruin' (Mrs Bear), 'Miss Chienne' (Miss Dog)
and 'Miss Renard' (Miss Fox) are a reference to the nature and origin
of their voluminous accessories and perhaps a sly suggestion as to the
characters of the women themselves.[4]

Unknown artist
'Male Dress 1791', published in the *Journal des Luxus und der Moden*,
Weimar, 1791

Hand-coloured etching, 19 × 11 cm
V&A: 29872:4

The *Journal des Luxus und der Moden* was the first German periodical
to include fashion plates, covering the latest fashions emerging in
France, England, Germany and Denmark. Its readers included the
nobility and the middle classes.[5] Here we see a young man dressed in
the English style (that is, the simple yet well-tailored clothes worn
by English aristocrats in the country). An issue published the same
year announced 'In male clothing one follows almost universally the
taste of the Englishman.'[6]

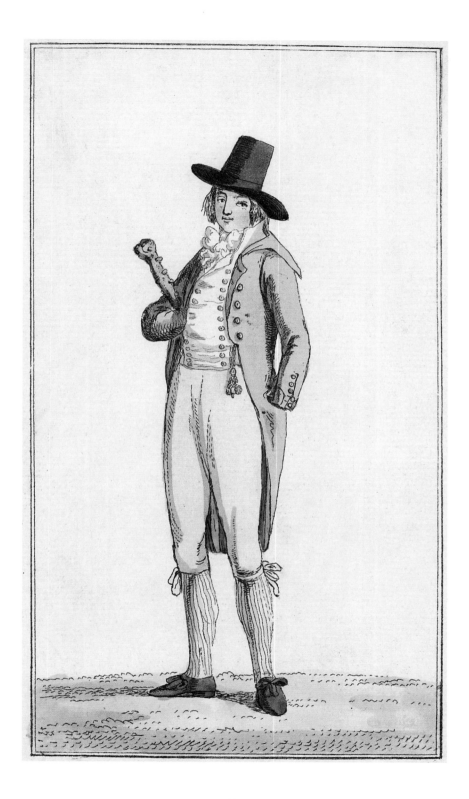

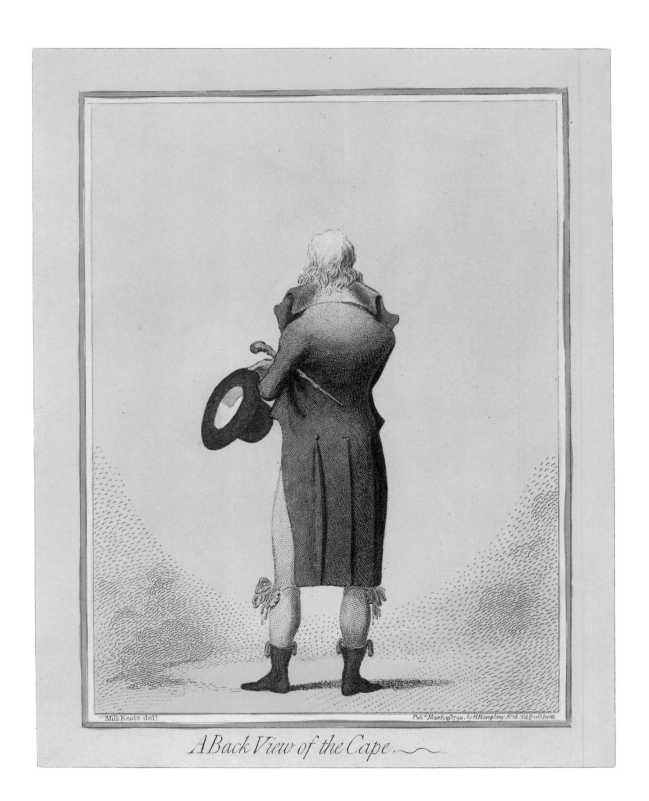

Mil: Keate del.

Pub.^d March 25 1792. by H.Humphrey N.o 8. Old Bond Street

A Back View of the Cape.

James Gillray (1756–1815), after Georgiana Keate (1770–1850)
'A Back View of the Cape.', published by Hannah Humphrey
(c.1745–1818), London, 23 March 1792

Hand-coloured etching, 28 × 22 cm
V&A: E.153–1989. Bequeathed by Frank A. Gibson.

Gillray delighted in taking fashion plates to task; this is one of two satirical prints he executed on the subject of men's high collars or 'capes', as they were then known.[7] The composition assumes the conventions of the fashion plate, in which figures were frequently portrayed from behind to show the cut and silhouette of their garments, with a lettered title beneath identifying the dress depicted. This 'Back View', however, reveals the considerable quantity of hair powder that has settled on the man's collar.

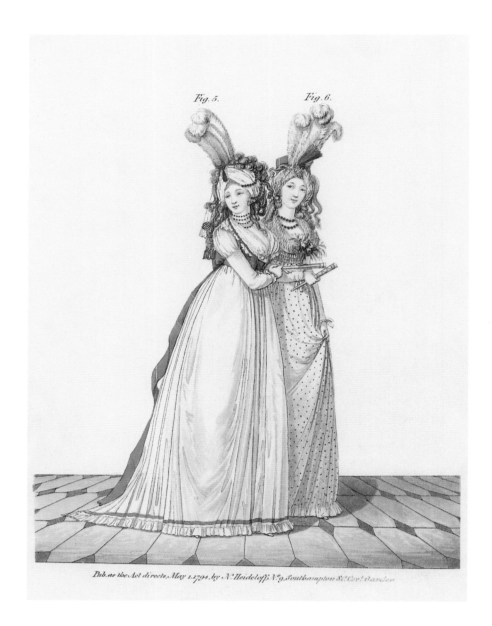

Fig. 5.   Fig. 6.

Pub. as the Act directe. May 1.1794. by N. Heideloff; N.º 9. Southampton St. Cov.t Garden

Nikolaus Wilhelm von Heideloff (1761–1837)
'Evening dresses', published in the *Gallery of Fashion*,
London, 1 May 1794

Hand-coloured etching and aquatint, 29 × 22.5 cm

National Art Library: RC.R.11

This charming scene is typical of the conviviality that characterized
the *Gallery of Fashion*. Heideloff's fashion plates excelled at evoking
a mood, usually through the judicious groupings of figures[8] and,
on occasion, the use of unusual perspectives and backdrops.[9] Both
women shown here wear headdresses *à la Turque*, described in the
accompanying text as turbans embellished with ostrich feathers,
pearls and other jewels. These lavish feathered headdresses were
irresistible to caricaturists, as Gillray's satire (opposite) shows.

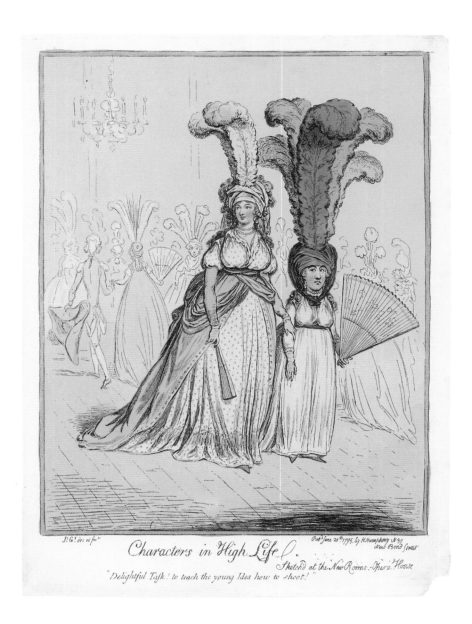

James Gillray (1756–1815)

**'Characters in High Life. Sketch'd at the New Rooms,
Opera House'**, published by Hannah Humphrey (c.1745–1818),
London, 20 June 1795

Hand-coloured etching, 36 × 27 cm
V&A: E.116–1989. Bequeathed by Frank A. Gibson.

The Duchess of Rutland, doyenne of fashionable Georgian society and
a celebrated beauty, is shown here as she appeared in several portraits
by Joshua Reynolds (1723–92), escorting her considerably less poised
companion, most likely one of her daughters, to the Theatre Royal
(known even then as the 'Opera House'), London.[10] Both women sport
the very latest in fashionable headwear – turbans ornamented with
vertiginous ostrich feathers, to which the punning title, 'Characters
in High Life', refers.

Horace Vernet (1789–1863)

'[no. 838] Capote de Paille Blanche. Costume Négligé.'
(White straw bonnet, undress [light or formal dress]),
published in the *Journal des dames et des modes*, Paris, 1807

Hand-coloured etching, 19.6 × 11.4 cm
Rueil-Malmaison, château de Malmaison et Bois-Préau

This informal morning ensemble includes the very latest in fashionable Regency headwear: a straw bonnet, commonly referred to as a 'poke' bonnet or 'coal-scuttle'. A fashion column in *The Times* of 1 December 1807 urged its readers to incorporate a 'poke bonnet of basket willow' into their morning walking attire.[11] In his manual on beauty and dress, however, the writer Auguste Caron was scathing on this 'barbarous kind of head-dress', remarking, not without irony, that it 'is attended with some advantages; it produces a very happy effect in caricatures, and some of our artists have not failed to avail themselves of it.'[12]

(838)

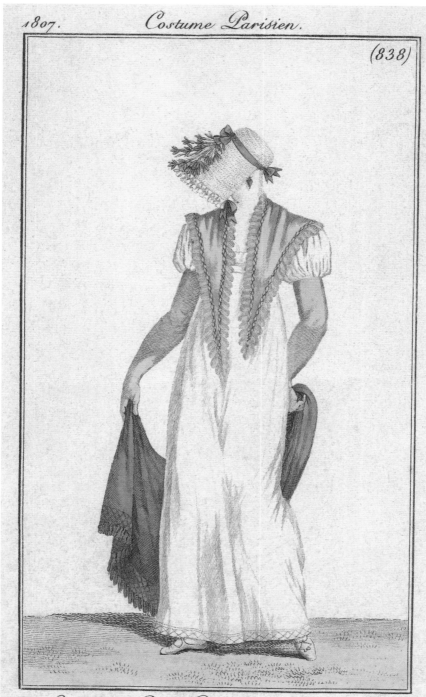

Capote de Paille Blanche. Costume Négligé.

James Gillray (1756–1815), after an anonymous French print
'Les Invisibles', published by Hannah Humphrey (*c*.1745–1818),
Paris and London, 1810

Hand-coloured etching, 23.8 × 31.2 cm
V&A: E.992–1970. Given by Major Nicholas Collin and Mr Francis Collin
at the request of their mother Mrs Frank Collin.

The French term for the Regency 'poke' bonnet was the 'invisible',
because the hat's deep peak shielded the wearer's face from view. Gillray
mocks both the fashion and those who modelled it – the fashionably
eccentric Parisian types, 'les incroyables' and 'les merveilleuses'. These
young men and women of Paris adopted outlandish ensembles in reaction
to the end of The Terror (the final, most violent phase of the French
Revolution). In satires, such figures were often depicted from behind,
or with their faces obscured, in imitation of their affected deportment,
which was also captured in contemporary fashion plates (previous page).

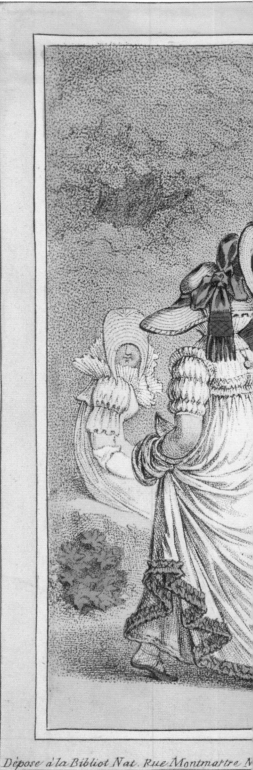

Déposé à la Bibliot Nat. Rue Montmartre N

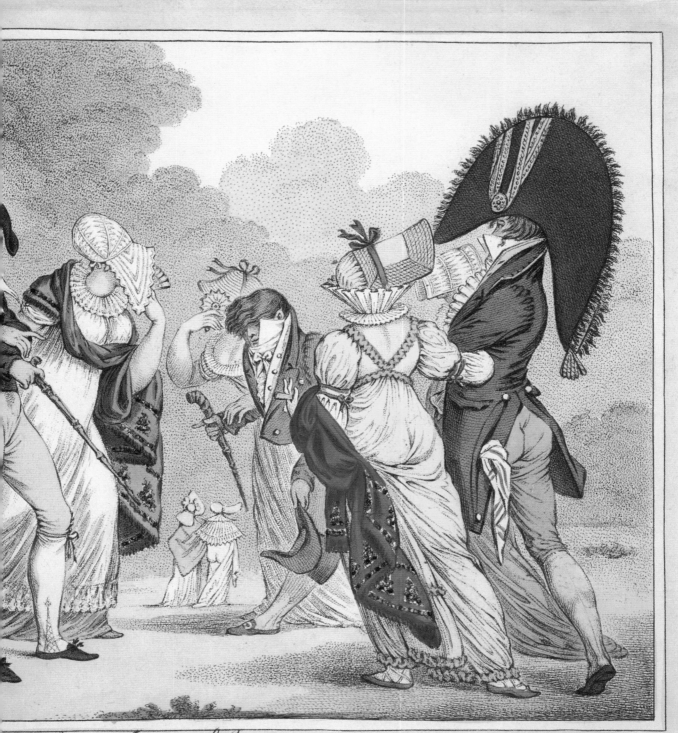

Les Invisibles . 1810 —   *et a Londrès, chez H. Humphrey . S.t James Street.*

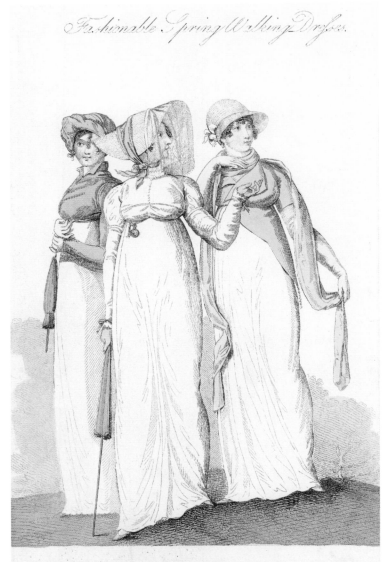

Fashionable Spring Walking Dresses.

aven for the 31st Number of La Belle Assemblee, Published on June 1.1808, for John Bell, proprietor of th
Messenger, Strand.

Unknown artist
'Fashionable Spring Walking Dresses', published in
La Belle Assemblée, London, June 1808

Hand-coloured etching, 21.8 × 13 cm
V&A: E.2456–1888

The high-waisted, diaphanous dresses of the early nineteenth century were intended to imitate the drapery seen in classical art. Fashion plates such as the one above emphasized this allusion by posing figures to evoke Greek and Roman sculptures. Looking back at fashion plates from the turn of the nineteenth century, Charles Baudelaire remarked that they 'can be translated into beauty or ugliness: in ugliness they become caricatures; in beauty, antique statues'.[13]

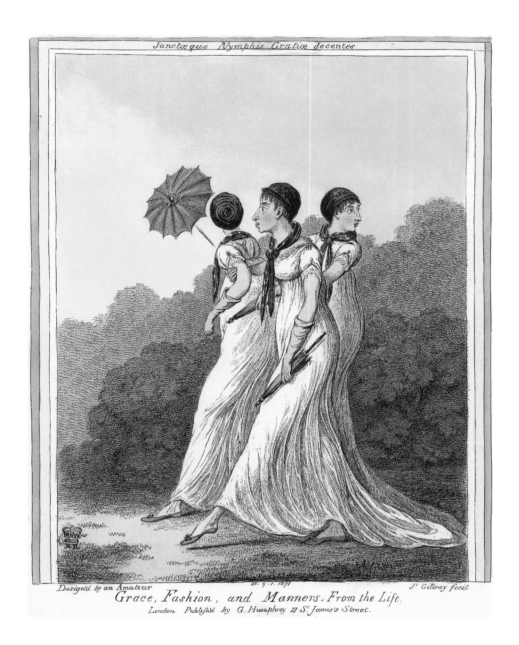

Junctæque Nymphis Gratiæ decentes

Design'd by an Amateur   *Js Gillray fecit*

Grace, Fashion, and Manners. From the Life.

London Publish'd by G. Humphrey 27 St James's Street.

James Gillray (1756–1815)

'Grace, Fashion and Manners. From the Life.',

published by Hannah Humphrey (*c.*1745–1818), London, 1810

Etching, 25.8 × 20 cm

British Museum

Both this and the satirical print overleaf (also on the classical theme of the 'Three Graces') play on the conventions of contemporary fashion plates, in which faces are usually generic and somewhat blank, thereby directing the reader's attention to the dress depicted and helping her to imagine herself in the place of the beautiful figure shown. Here, by contrast, the faces are caricatures of three well-known women of Regency England (the daughters of Sir William Manners).

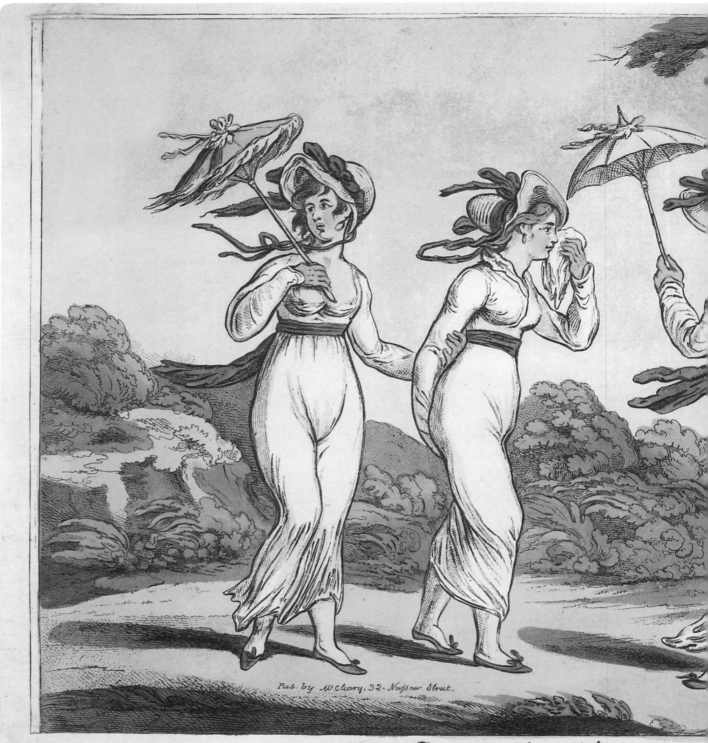

Pub. by W. Cleary, 32. Nassau Street.

The GRACES in a high Wind

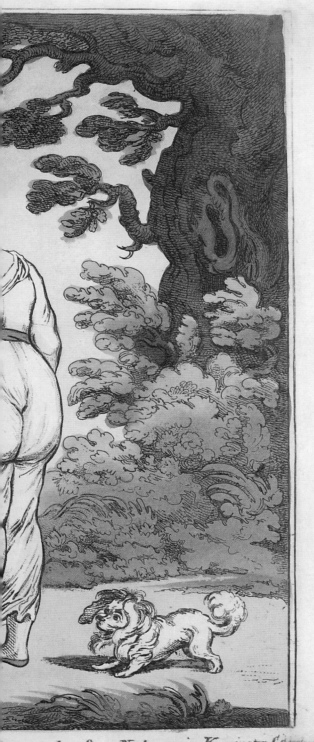

cene taken from Nature, in Kensington G...

Unknown printmaker, after James Gillray (1756–1815)

'The Graces in a high Wind – a Scene taken from Nature, in Kensington Gardens', published by McLeary, Dublin, 1810

Hand-coloured etching, 24.1 × 34.3 cm
V&A: E.510–1955. Given by Mr Geoffrey A. Whittall.

Gillray's satire references the artistic tradition of depicting the 'Three Graces' of classical mythology (in which one of the figures is, by convention, shown from behind) to mock the classicizing pretensions of fashion plates such as those found in *La Belle Assemblée*. Figures in fashion plates generally gaze gently into the distance without looking at each other or engaging with the gaze of the viewer – safely unobserved, the viewer can, therefore, indulge in the pleasure of looking. Gillray exaggerates the obliviousness of his 'Graces', and the voyeurism their dress invites.

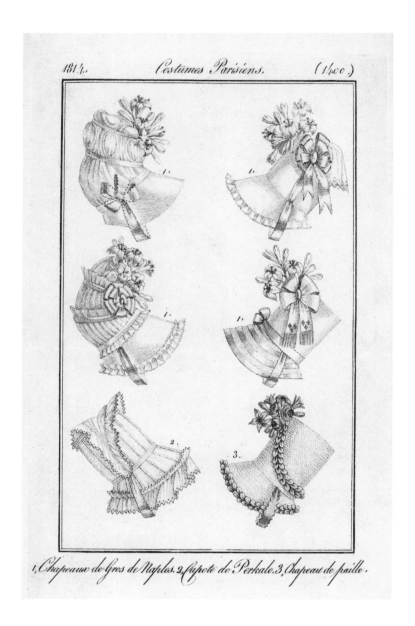

1, Chapeaux de Gros de Naples. 2, Capote de Perkale. 3, Chapeau de paille.

Unknown artist, possibly Horace Vernet (1789–1863)
**'[no. 1400] 1. Chapeaux de Gros de Naples. 2. Capote de Perkale.
3. Chapeau de paille.' (1. Plain weave Italian silk hats.
2. Percale cotton bonnet. 3. Straw hat.)**, published in the
Journal des dames et des modes, Paris, 1815

Hand-coloured etching, 19.6 × 11.4 cm
Private collection

The Vernets were something of a fashion dynasty – Horace Vernet's
grandfather, Jean-Michel Moreau 'le jeune', was responsible for the
elegant illustrations to the *Monument du costume* (1775–83, p.14), and
his father, Carle Vernet (1758–1835), also produced fashion plates for
the highly influential *Journal des dames et des modes*. The magazine
appeared every five days and could therefore rightly claim to record the
very latest fashions from Paris. This plate shows the highly decorated
bonnets, with exaggeratedly tall crowns, favoured by the 'merveilleuses'.

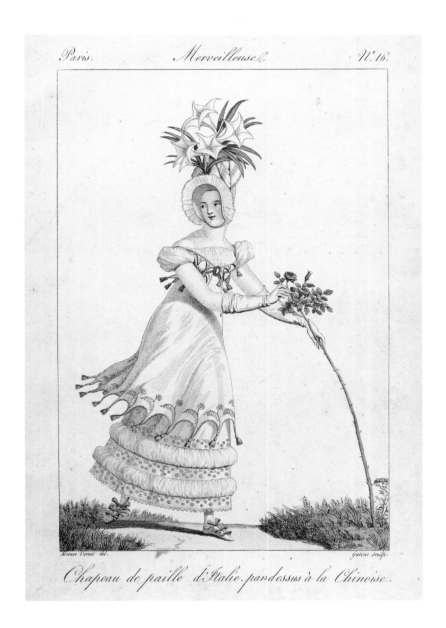

Horace Vernet del.   *Gatine sculp.*

Chapeau de paille d'Italie, par-dessus à la Chinoise.

Georges Jacques Gatine (1773–*c.*1841), after Horace Vernet (1789–1863)
'Merveilleuse: Chapeau de paille d'Italie, par-dessus à la Chinoise.'
(Merveilleuse: Italian straw hat, overdress in the Chinese style.),
no.16 from the series *Incroyables et Merveilleuses* (1810–1818),
published by Pierre de La Mésangère (1759–1831), Paris, *c.*1813

Hand-coloured etching, 37 × 25 cm

V&A: E.133–1947

Pierre de La Mésangère commissioned this deluxe series of 33 large,
hand-coloured plates for his *Journal des dames et des modes* and it was
clearly designed to amuse; an 1812 issue of the *Journal* announced
that there would be a delay in the issue of the next plate in the series,
as the existing satire had been judged insufficiently exaggerated.[14]
So eccentric were the real-life fashions of 'incroyables' and 'merveilleuses',
however, that audiences were divided as to whether the series
constituted fashion plates or satires.

Unknown artist
'Walking Dress.', published in *La Belle Assemblée*,
London, September 1822

Hand-coloured etching, 26.8 × 16.5 cm
V&A: E.2818–1888

A month after this fashion plate was published, George Cruikshank included an almost identical ensemble in his satirical print 'Monstrosities of 1822' (overleaf). He may well have used the plate as a direct source for the contemporary fashion detail. Compare the tightly belted green and purple-check dress, plumed hat and protruding slipper, illustrated here, with the female figure on the far right of Cruikshank's print.

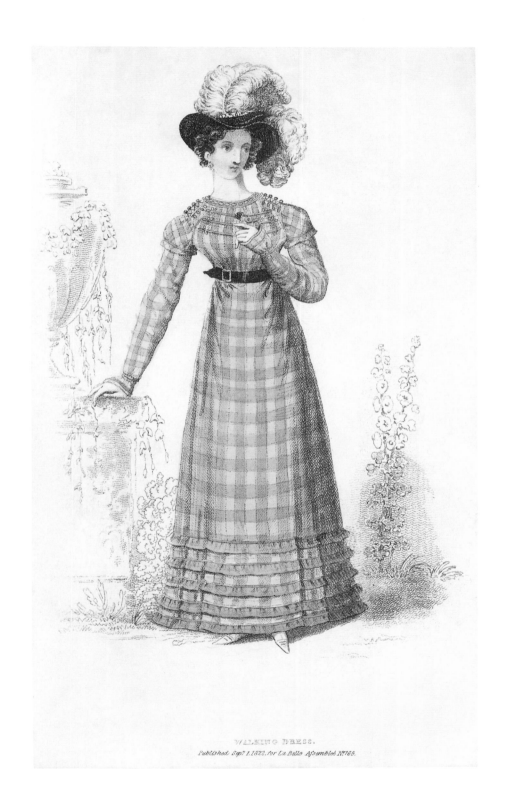

WALKING DRESS.
Published Sep! 1, 1822, for La Belle Assemblée N°165.

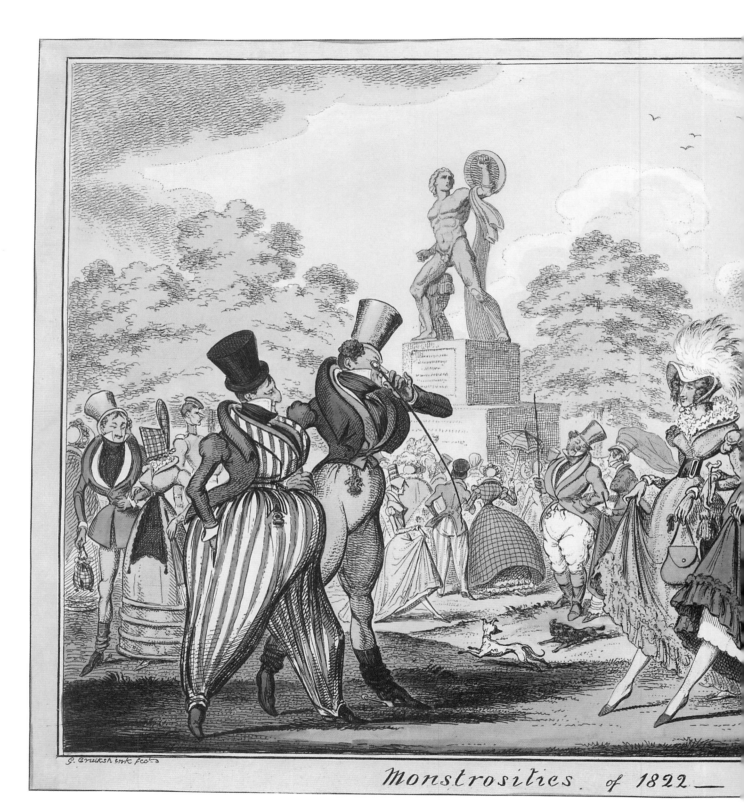

Monstrosities. of 1822.

G. Cruiksh^{ank} fec.^t

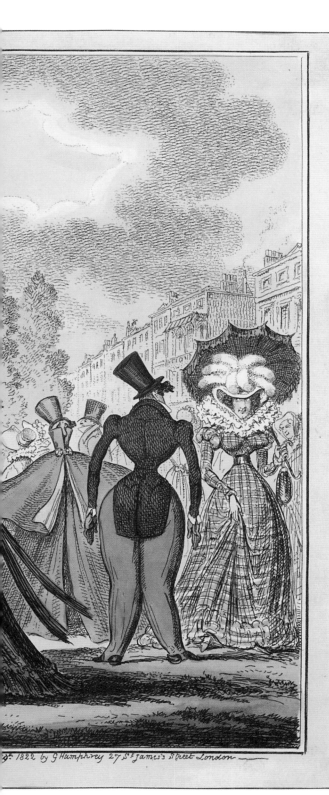

George Cruikshank (1792–1878)
'Monstrosities of 1822', published by G. Humphrey,
London, 19 October 1822

Hand-coloured etching, 26.5 × 36.6 cm
V&A: 9481.C. Given by Mrs George Cruikshank.

The fashionable crowd, gathered to promenade in London's parks, were
the perfect subject for the satirist looking to explore contemporary dress.
Here, the classically proportioned statue of Achilles (a real sculpture,
by Richard Westmacott, unveiled in Hyde Park a few months before the
print was published) is used to highlight the constricting, flamboyant
nature of the garments worn below. Cruikshank published his
'Monstrosities' prints, all set in Hyde Park, annually between 1818 and
1827, satirizing the fashions of the preceding year. As this example
demonstrates, they were packed with accurate details of fabrics,
trimmings and accessories.

Unknown artist
'Parisian Ball Dress.', published by Joseph Robins (*fl.*1820–40),
London and Dublin, 1 May 1827

Hand-coloured steel engraving, 15 × 9.5 cm
V&A: E.2340–1888

A young woman wearing a pink silk ball dress in the 'Parisian' – for which, read the 'latest' – style assumes a graceful pose, lifting her skirt to reveal her elegant ankle and a neat pair of dancing slippers. The focal point of the print, however, is her dramatic hairstyle, known as an 'Apollo's Knot' and described in a November 1827 issue of *La Belle Assembleé* as 'a row of large puffs of hair'[15] – false hair worn over wire loops.[16] These loops were usually further ornamented with the addition of ribbons and flowers, only increasing the girth of the coiffure.

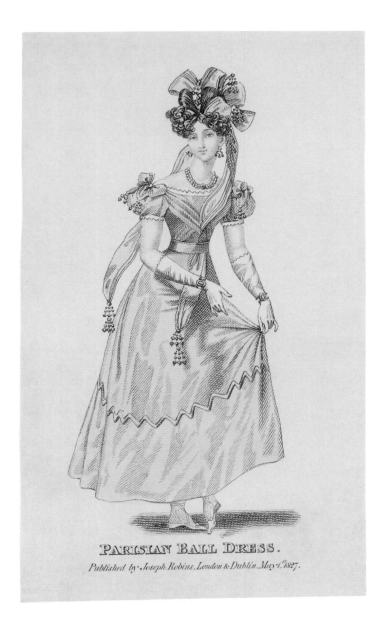

PARISIAN BALL DRESS.

Published by Joseph Robins, London & Dublin, May 1st 1827.

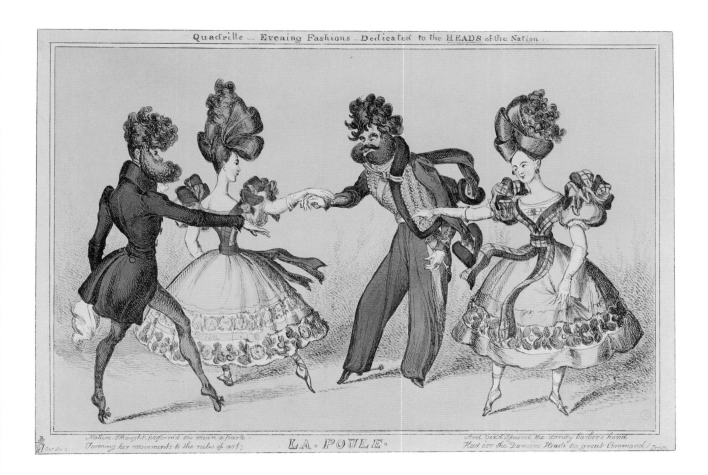

Quadrille – Evening Fashions – Dedicated to the HEADS of the Nation.

Nature I thought, perform'd too mean a parte
Forming her movements to the rules of art;

LA. POULE.

And vex'd I found the dandy barbers hand
Had o'er the Dancers Heads too great Command.

William Heath (1795–1840)

'La Poule. Quadrille – Evening Fashions – Dedicated to the HEADS of the Nation', published by Thomas McLean (1788–1875), London, 1827

Hand-coloured etching, 25.5 × 37 cm

V&A: 23689:7. Townshend Bequest.

Heath casts a critical eye over the hairstyles of his time in this print, in which two dandies lead their partners in the quadrille, a popular French dance. Heath exaggerates the women's 'Apollo's Knot' hairstyles and their fashionably short ball dresses. The title, 'La Poule', evokes the farmyard strut of the hen and her mate. The verse underneath reads 'And vex'd I found the dandy barbers hand/ Had o'er the Dancers Heads too great Command'.

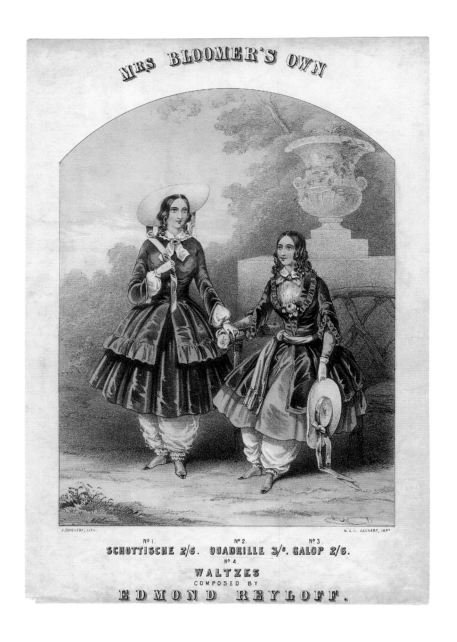

J. Coventry (lithographer)
'Mrs Bloomer's Own', mass-produced
lithographic song sheet, *c*.1850

Lithograph on paper, 34.5 × 24.1 cm
V&A: S.345–2012. Gabrielle Enthoven Collection.

In North America, in the 1850s, there was a movement to reform women's dress by replacing long skirts with a form of pantaloon or baggy trouser. These experimental garments were popularly known as 'Bloomers' after Mrs Amelia Jenks Bloomer, a women's rights campaigner who was one of their chief advocates. The design of bloomers aimed to retain a feminine appearance. They therefore took inspiration, not from men's trousers, but from female Turkish costume and children's dress.

WOMAN'S EMANCIPATION.

(Being a Letter addressed to Mr. Punch, with a Drawing, by a strong-minded American Woman.)

It is quite easy to realise the considerable difficulty that the natives of this old country are like to have in estimating the rapid progress of ideas on all subjects among us, the Anglo-Saxons of the Western World. Mind travels with us on a rail-car, or a high-pressure river-boat. The snags and sawyers of prejudice, which render so dangerous the navigation of Time's almighty river, whose water-power has toppled over these giant-growths of the world, without being able to detach them from the congenial mud from which they draw their nutriment, are dashed aside or run down in the headlong career of the United States mind.

We laugh to scorn the dangers of popular effervescence. Our almighty-browed and cavernous-eyed statesmen sit, heroically, on the safety-valve, and the mighty ark of our vast Empire of the West moves on at a pressure on the square inch which would rend into shivers the rotten boiler-plates of your outworn states of the Old World.

To use a phrase, which the refined manners of our ladies have banished from the drawing-room, and the saloon of the boarding-house, *we* go a-head. And our progress is the progress of all—not of high and low, for we have abolished the odious distinction—but of man, woman, and child, each in his or her several sphere.

Our babies are preternaturally sharp, and highly independent from the cradle. The high-souled American boy will not submit to be whipped at school. That punishment is confined to negroes and the lower animals.

But it is among *our* sex—among women—(for I am a woman, and my name is Theodosia Eudoxia Bang, of Boston, U.S., Principal of the Homœopathic and Collegiate Thomsonian Institute for developing the female mind in that intellectual city)—that the stranger may realise in the most convincing manner the progressional influences of the democratic institutions it is our privilege to live under.

An American female—for I do not like the term Lady, which suggests the outworn distinctions of feudalism—can travel alone from one end of the States to the other—from the majestic waters of Niagara to the mystic banks of the Yellow-stone, or the rolling prairies of Texas. The American female delivers lectures—edits newspapers, and similar organs of opinion, which exert so mighty a leverage on the national mind of our great people—is privileged to become a martyr to her principles, and to utter her soul from the platform, by the side of the gifted Poe or the immortal Peabody. All this in these old countries is the peculiar privilege of man, as opposed to woman. The female is consigned to the slavish duties of the house. In America the degrading cares of the household are comparatively unknown to our sex. The American wife resides in a boarding-house, and, consigning the petty cares of daily life to the helps of the establishment, enjoys leisure for higher pursuits, and can follow her vast aspirations upwards, or in any other direction.

We are emancipating ourselves, among other badges of the slavery of feudalism, from the inconvenient dress of the European female. With man's functions, we have asserted our right to his garb, and especially to that part of it which invests the lower extremities. With this great symbol, we have adopted others,—the hat, the cigar, the paletot or round jacket. And it is generally calculated that the dress of the Emancipated American female is quite pretty,—as becoming in all points as it is manly and independent. I enclose a drawing made by my gifted fellow-citizen, Increasen Tarbox, of Boston, U.S., for the *Free Woman's Banner*, a periodical under my conduct, aided by several gifted women of acknowledged progressive opinions.

I appeal to my sisters of the Old World, with confidence, for their sympathy and their countenance in the struggle in which *we* are engaged, and which will soon be found among them also. For I feel that I have a mission across the broad Atlantic, and the steamers are now running at reduced fares. I hope to rear the standard of Female Emancipation on the roof of the Crystal Palace in London Hyde Park. Empty wit may sneer at its form, which is bifurcate. And why not? Mahomet warred under the Petticoat of his wife Kadiga. The American female Emancipist marches on her holy war under the distinguishing garment of her husband. In the compartment devoted to the United States in your Exposition, my sisters of the old country may see this banner by the side of a uniform of female freedom,—such as my drawing represents,—the garb of martyrdom for a month; the trappings of triumph for all ages of the future!

Theodosia E. Bang, M.A.,
M.C.P., Φ.Δ.Κ., K.L.M., &c., &c., (of Boston, U.S.).

John Tenniel (1820–1914)

'WOMAN'S EMANCIPATION. (Being a Letter addressed to Mr. Punch, with a Drawing, by a strong-minded American Woman)', published in *Punch*, London, 5 July 1851

Wood engraving, 10.6 × 17.7 cm

National Art Library: PP.8.H–L

Although never widely adopted in mainstream society, the very idea of bloomers as a replacement for long skirts provoked severe censure. This had less to do with the erotic potential of revealing women's legs than the fear of women appropriating male dress and, by extension, male power and privilege. The skirts worn over bloomers actually fell below the knee but, in this *Punch* cartoon, they look more like the frock coats conventionally worn by Victorian men. The cartoon makes an explicit connection between 'bloomerism' and campaigns for women's rights.

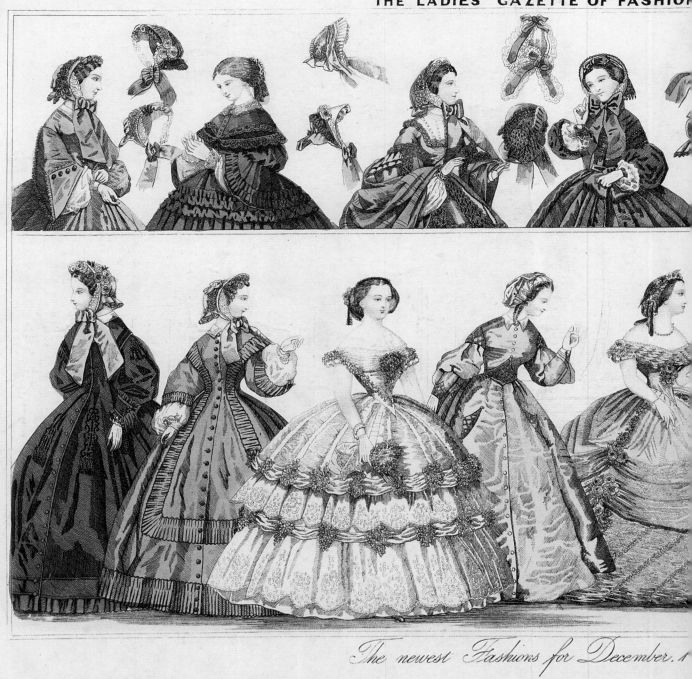

The newest Fashions for December. 1

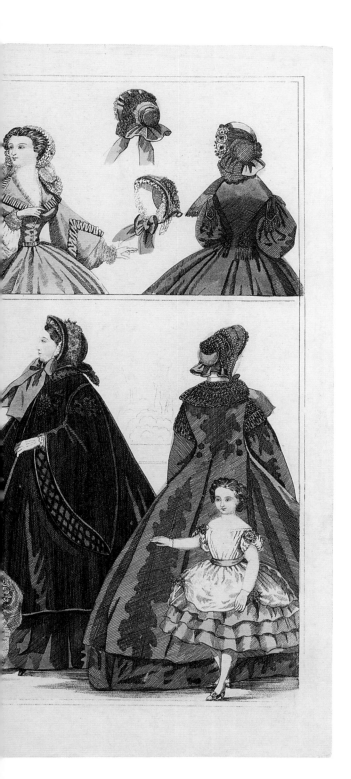

Unknown artist
'The newest Fashions for December 1860.', published in
The Ladies' Gazette of Fashion, London, December 1860

Hand-coloured lithograph, 38 × 53.5 cm
V&A: E.2229–1934. Given by Colonel G. Morphew.

Women's skirts had reached exaggerated proportions by the early 1860s.
The style was achieved by means of a crinoline – a structure of spring-
steel hoops worn under the skirt to support and distend the fabric.
The figures in this fashion plate are carefully spread across a double
page, emphasizing the stately presence of the garments and the amount
of space they occupied. This plate also promotes the sensory pleasures
of fashion: the women feel the fabric of their clothing and the hand-
colouring of the print replicates the intense hues made possible in
this period by the development of new synthetic fabric dyes.

W. Brandard (*fl.*mid-nineteenth century)
'Song for Leap Year, The Ladies' Opportunity!
Dedicated to the Young Ladies of England. by E.T. Wattson
and Carlo Minasi, London', published by Stannard & Dixon,
London, *c.*1860

Colour lithograph, 35 × 25 cm
Michael Diamond Collection

The crinoline was satirized obsessively, across all forms of popular print.
A favourite theme was the disruption to domestic harmony caused by
crinolines, because of their cost, their size and the implication that they
kept men at arms length. Positing that crinolines had no use value,
satirists came up with many ways in which they might be appropriated
– as fire guards or bathing machines for example. Here, women use a
crinoline as a cage to trap a man, in a pun on the leap year referenced
in the title – when a woman was traditionally allowed to overturn the
social order by proposing marriage to a man.

SONG FOR LEAP YEAR,
THE LADIES' OPPORTUNITY !

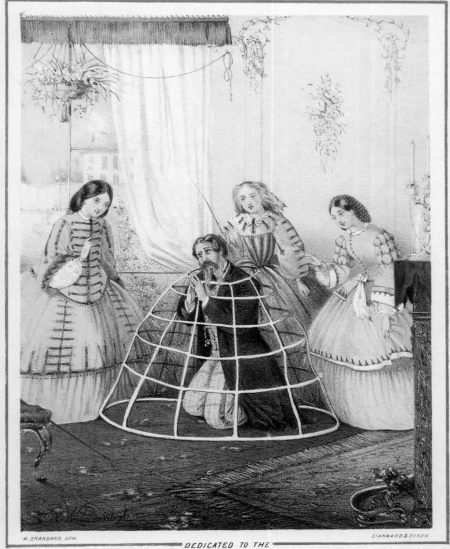

W. BRANDARD, LITH.

STANNARD & DIXON

DEDICATED TO THE
YOUNG LADIES OF ENGLAND.
BY
E. T. WATTSON AND CARLO MINASI,

ENT. STA HALL

Pr: 2/6

LONDON;

METZLER & Cº 37, 39 & 38, Gt MARLBOROUGH ST W

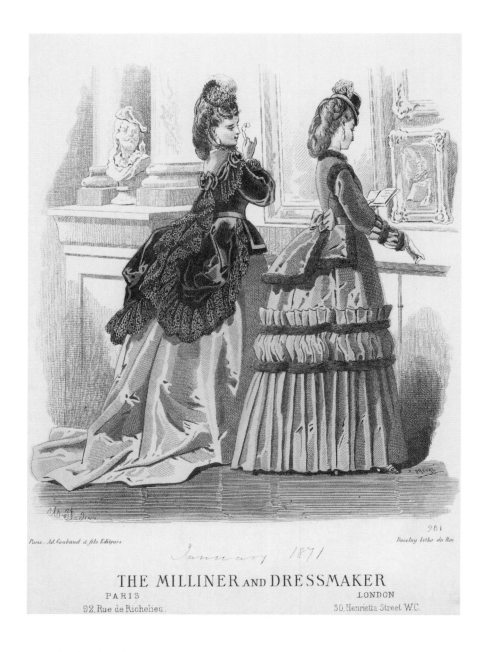

THE MILLINER AND DRESSMAKER

PARIS   LONDON

92, Rue de Richelieu.   30, Henrietta Street, W.C.

Amédée Bodin (1825–*c.*1871), after E. Préval (*fl.*mid-nineteenth century)
Untitled, published in *The Milliner and Dressmaker*,
London, January 1871

Hand-coloured litho-engraving, 31.8 × 19.7 cm

V&A: E.1878–1888

Fashion plate illustrators of this period drew figures interacting in
detailed social settings, bringing the prints closer in form to the mild
social satires of upper-middle-class life that also appeared in smart
magazines. The backdrop is often a sumptuous home or public place
with cultural prestige. Here, two women admire a female portrait in
an art gallery, all the while making a picture of themselves by displaying
their fashionable silhouettes.

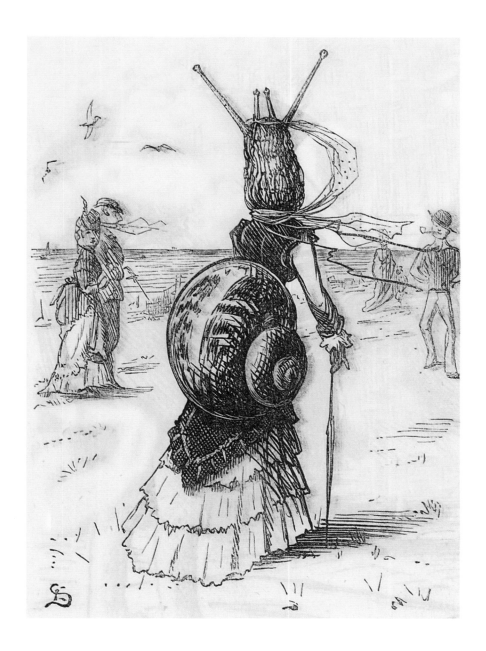

Linley Sambourne (1844–1910)
Untitled, published in *Punch*, London, 1870

Wood engraving, 10 × 7.4 cm
V&A: E.475–2010. Given by Catherine Flood.

By 1870, the fashionable silhouette for women was curvaceous – padded out at the back with a structured undergarment called a bustle. In this print, Linley Sambourne humorously suggests that this garment changes the female form by means of a kind of backwards evolution – the woman is turning into a snail. This was the period in which Charles Darwin was unfolding his theory of evolution, and its implications for science and society were hotly debated.

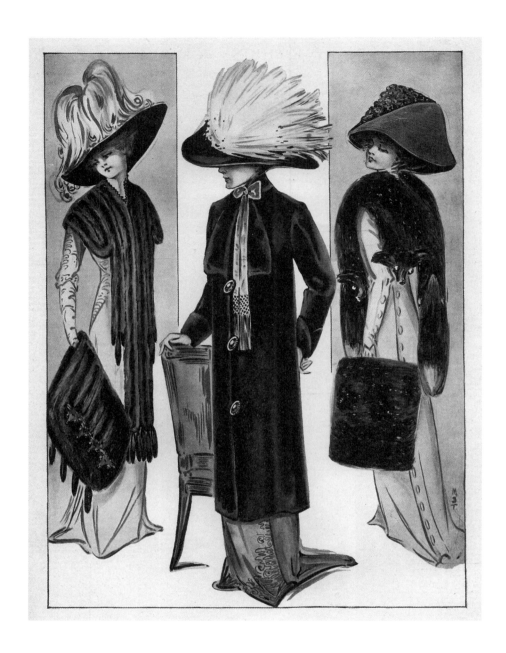

Unidentified artist, signed 'MCT'
'Midwinter Fashions in Fur from the Plymouth Fur Company',
published in *Vogue*, New York, 11 December 1909

Process print, dimensions unknown
The Vogue Archive

The first decade of the twentieth century saw the emerging world of haute couture embrace fur, which began to feature prominently in seasonal collections. Full-length coats where fur was used as a key material, rather than as a lining, were an innovation of this period and became one of fashion's most prominent symbols of luxury and wealth. The use of fur on accessories – particularly muffs, stoles and hats – added to the impression that the wearer was enveloped in fur.

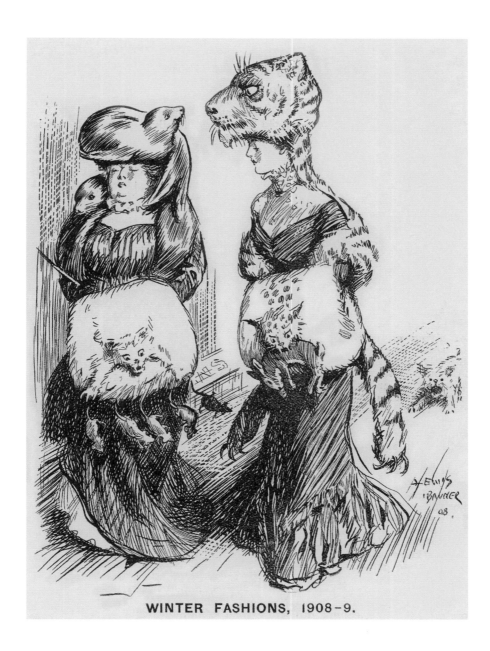

WINTER FASHIONS, 1908-9.

Lewis Baumer (1870–1963)
'Winter Fashions, 1908–9.', published in *Punch*,
London, 9 December 1908

Line block print, 16.8 × 12 cm
National Art Library: PP.8.H-L

From the 1890s, fur muffs and stoles were often decorated with
the heads and tails of the animals whose skins had been used.
The winter of 1908–9 was notable for a similar treatment being
applied to enormous hats, a trend that is burlesqued in the *Punch*
cartoon above. Rather than being elegantly draped, the (unusual)
selection of animals appears alert and alive, even going so far
as to capture furry prey.

Fernand Siméon (1884–1928)

'Le Retour des autans: Tailleur et Robe d'après-midi, de Dœuillet' (The Return of the Southerly Winds: Suit and afternoon dress by Dœuillet), published in the *Gazette du Bon Ton*, Paris, September 1920

Pochoir, 24.6 × 19 cm
V&A: CIRC.122–1975

Two elegant women model autumnal ensembles designed by celebrated couturier Georges Dœuillet (1865–1929). The silhouette has changed, from the fussy volume of the Edwardian period to the more streamlined and unstructured 'barrel-line' adopted by liberated women of the 1920s. The fashion plate itself has also changed to embrace a more graphic aesthetic and a more pronounced mood and attitude.

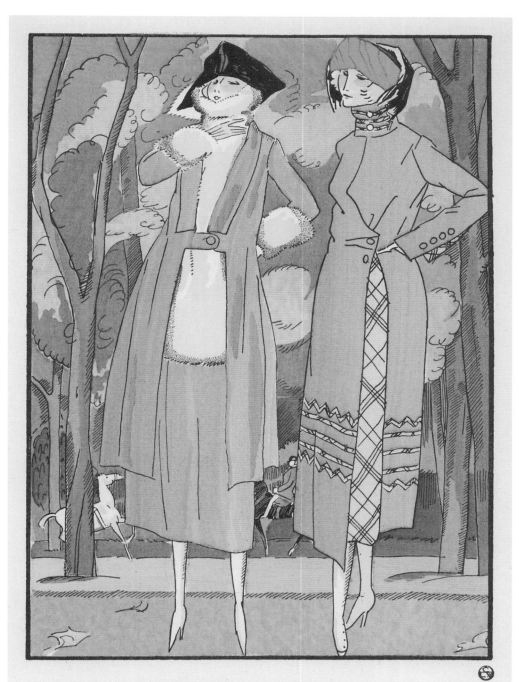

LE RETOUR DES AUTANS

Tailleur et Robe d'après-midi, de Dœuillet

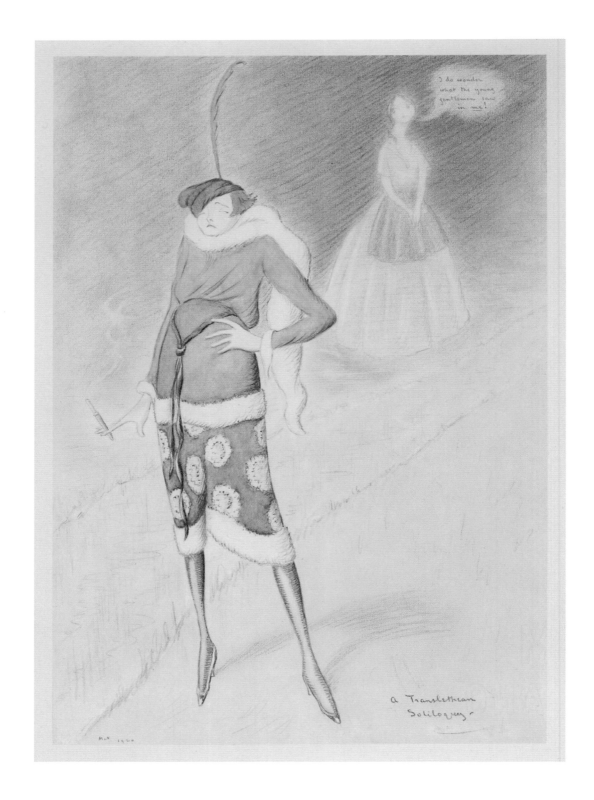

Henry Maximilian [Max] Beerbohm (1872–1956)
'A Translethean Soliloquy – "I do wonder what the young gentlemen saw in *me!*", England, 1920

Watercolour, 53 × 37.4 cm
V&A: CIRC.996–1967

The young woman in this watercolour (which was probably intended for publication) represents the essence of 1920s modernity, with her short hemline, elegantly held cigarette and imperious demeanour. Her angular posture and elongated legs mirror those of the figures in stylized fashion plates of her time (previous page). She would be unrecognizable to her forebears, embodied by the demure young woman of the 1840s, 'A Damsel of the 'Keepsake' Time', who is seen in the background. The river Lethe – in Greek mythology, the river of forgetfulness – is used to emphasize how fashion had changed over the past 80 years.

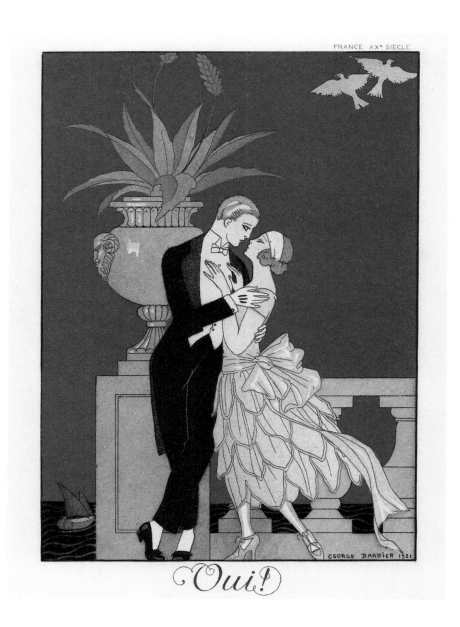

George Barbier (1882–1932)

'Oui!', published in *Falbalas et fanfreluches: Almanach des modes
présentes, passées et futures*, Paris, 1922 (designed 1921)

Process engraving and *pochoir*, 20.7 × 14.2 cm
V&A: C.6694:1

The most common technique used for 1920s fashion plates was *pochoir*,
a form of hand-stencilling that used luminous shades of watercolour
– each colour painted through a cut stencil – to communicate the
freshness and vivacity of the Art Deco aesthetic. Barbier created many
such plates for the luxury publications of his day, including *Falbalas
et fanfreluches*. He often grouped his figures to suggest a narrative –
in this scene, an ecstatic but enigmatic 'Yes!' issues from the amorous
young couple on the balcony.

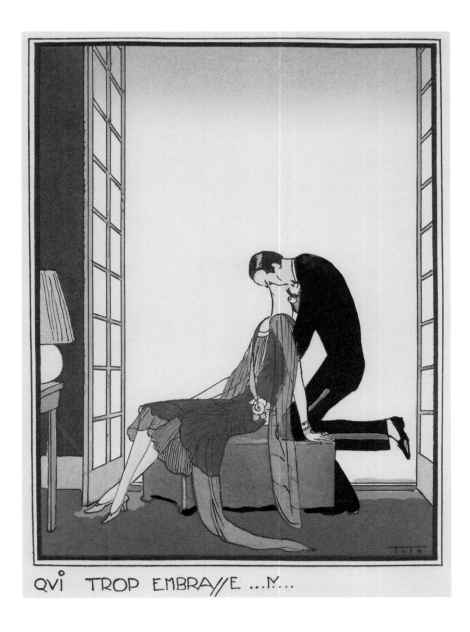

QVI TROP EMBRA//E ...M...

Ettore Tito (1859–1941)

'Qui trop embrasse…' (He who embraces too much...),
from the series *Quatre Proverbes*, published in Paris, 1927

Line block-coloured by hand, 20.3 × 15.2 cm
V&A: E.898–1975. Given by Mr and Mrs L.H. Urry.

Tito spoofs the highly-stylized Art Deco fashion plates of his time, which paired scenes of improbably elegant couples with obscure captions. He also gives a licentious veneer to the romantic scenarios beloved of fashion plate illustrators. The caption hints at the French proverb 'Qui trop embrasse mal étreint' (He who embraces too much, grasps nothing) and is applied here to the wandering hands of the young man, which are just discernible under the woman's transparent dress. This may also be a wry commentary on the trend for a flat-chested silhouette.

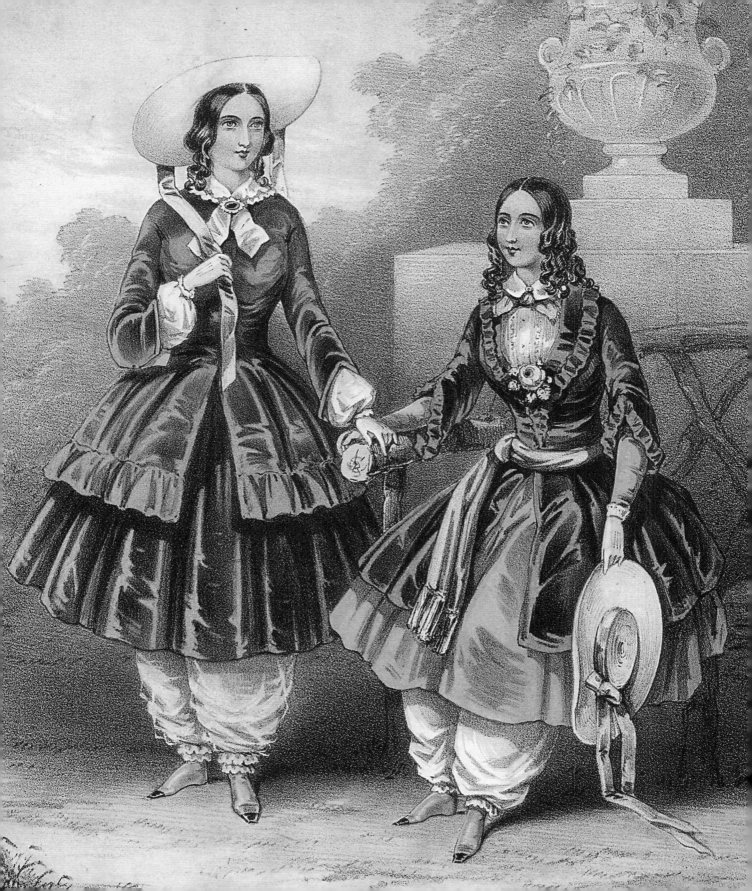

NOTES

AUTHORS' NOTE

1. Holland 1988, p.35
2. Vyvyan Holland wrote 'the best public collection of fashion magazines is, without question, in the Victoria and Albert Museum'; Holland 1988, p.163. Sir George Trenchard Cox, Director of the Museum from 1955 to 1966 declared it 'one of the finest' in the world; 'Foreword', Gibbs-Smith 1960.

STYLE AND SATIRE: CREATING FASHION FANTASIES

1. Sharon Marcus, *Between Women: Friendship, Desire and Marriage in Victorian England* (New York 2007), p.117
2. Valerie Steele, 'Art and Fashion', http://bit.ly/PwO88c, accessed 12 March 2014
3. Charles Baudelaire, *The Painter of Modern Life* (London 2010), p.14. First published 1863 in *Figaro*.
4. Ibid., p.5
5. Sheila O'Connell, *The Popular Print in England* (London 1999), p.11
6. *La Belle Assemblée* (June 1810), vol. 1, p.246
7. See Ralph Hyde and Valerie Cumming, 'The Prints of Benjamin Read, Tailor and Printmaker', *Print Quarterly* (September 2000), vol. 17, no. 3, pp.262–4. Compare George Cruikshank, 'Monstrosities of 1827', with Benjamin Read, 'Summer, a view in Hyde Park' (1827).
8. Ribeiro 1995, p.76
9. Ibid., p.3
10. Godfrey 1984, p.15
11. Robert Darnton, *The Forbidden Best-Sellers of Pre-Revolutionary France* (New York and London 1996), p.200
12. Rachel Jacobs, *Playing, Learning, Flirting: Printed Board Games from 18th Century France*, exh. pamphlet, Waddeson Manor (Waddeson 2012)
13. *An Exhibition in Honour of the Bicentenary of William Hogarth 1697–1764*, exh. cat., British Museum, London (London 1965), p.5
14. Bianca M. du Mortier, 'Fashion in Prints', *Print Quarterly*, vol. 7, no. 3, 1990, p.324
15. Nevinson 1967, p.84
16. See Gaudriault 1983 for a comprehensive survey of this development.
17. Holland 1988, p.35
18. Daniel Roche, *The culture of clothing: dress and fashion in the 'ancien régime'* (Cambridge 1994), p.477
19. Anne Buck and Harry Matthews, 'Pocket Guides to Fashion: Ladies' Pocket Books Published in England, 1760–1830', *Costume* (1984), no. 18, p.35
20. Gaudriault 1983, p.34
21. *Le Cabinet des modes* continued as *Le Magasin des modes nouvelles françaises et anglaises* (1786–9) and, subsequently, as *Le Journal de la mode du gout* (1790–3).
22. Roche (cited note 18), p.471
23. '& généralement de tout ce que la Mode offre de singulier, d'agréable ou d'intéressant dans tous les genres.', *Le Cabinet des modes* (1 January 1786), vol. 4, p.25 (frontispiece)
24. Roche (cited note 18), p.471
25. *La Belle Assemblée or Bell's Court and Fashionable Magazine*, vol. 1, part 1, February 1806
26. 'Advertisement', *Gallery of Fashion* (1794), vol. I, pp.1–2
27. Elisabeth-Louise Vigée Le Brun, *Elisabeth Vigée-Lebrun, Memoirs of a Painter: An Extraordinary Life Before, During and After the French Revolution* (Coventry 2009), p.13
28. Fiona Ffoulkes, '"Quality always distinguishes itself": Louis Hippolyte Le royal and the luxury clothing industry in early nineteenth century Paris', *Consumers and luxury: Consumer culture in Europe 1650–1850* (Manchester and New York 1999), p.184
29. See Robert Dighton, 'A Windy Day, scene outside the shop of Bowles the printseller' (c.1785, V&A: D.843–1900), James Gillray's 'Very slippy weather' (1808, V&A: 1232:44–1882), and J. Elwood, 'A crowd outside a printshop' (1790, British Museum).
30. Godfrey 1984, p.33
31. Holland 1988, p.162
32. For more on these practices, see M. A. Ghering van Ierlant, *Mode in Print (1550–1914)* (The Hague 1988).
33. Arlene Leis, 'Displaying Art and Fashion: Ladies' Pocket-Book Imagery in the Paper Collections of Sarah Sophia Banks', *Konsthistorisk Tidskrift* (22 August 2013), vol. 82, no. 3
34. Catherine M. Sama, 'Liberty, Equality, Frivolity! An Italian Critique of Fashion Periodicals', *Eighteenth-Century Studies* (2004), vol. 37, no. 3, p.392
35. Roche (cited note 18), p.143
36. Cited in Brian Dolan, *Ladies of the Grand Tour* (London 2001), p.179
37. Ibid., p.178
38. W.H. Wyatt, *The Lady's Toilette; Containing a Critical Examination of the Nature of Beauty… An Historical Sketch of the Fashions of France and England, etc.* (London 1808), p.34
39. Ibid., p.35

40. Frances Burney, *Camilla: Or, a picture of youth* (London 1802), p.127

41. Anonymous, *A fashionable caricature, or The proverbs of our ancestors* (London 1792), up.

42. Valerie Steele, 'The Social and Political Significance of Macaroni Fashion', *Costume 19* (1985), p.96

43. 'A letter from "A Southern Faunist" to "Mr Urban" on the yeomanry "notwithstanding it is hard in these days to exactly define what a yeoman or farmer really is"', *The Gentleman's Magazine and Historical Chronicle* (July 1801), vol. 71, part two, p.589

44. Caitlin Blackwell, '"The Feather'd Fair in a Fright": The Emblem of the Feather in Graphic Satire of 1776', *Journal for Eighteenth Century Studies* (September 2013), vol. 36, no. 3, pp.353–76

45. *Englishwoman's Domestic Magazine, Figure Training or Art the Handmaid of Nature* (London 1871), p.17

46. Anonymous, *The Whole Art of the Dress! Or, the Road to Elegance and Fashion At the Enormous Saving of Thirty Per Cent!!!* (London 1830), p.6

47. Godfrey 1984, p.33

48. A.E. Johnson, *Dudley Hardy* (London 1909), p.40

49. See Beetham 1996.

50. Eliza Lynn Linton, 'The Girl of the Period', *The Saturday Review* (14 March 1868), vol. 25, no. 646, pp.339–40

51. See the print 'Latest Fashions', *Punch* (1870), vol. 59, p.221.

52. Pencil inscription to the engraver on Jules David, untitled fashion plate design (1866, V&A: E.13–1966).

53. The Colin sisters were Héloïse (1820–75), Anaïs (1822–99), Laure (1820–78) and Isabelle (1850–1907). See Kyriaki Hadjiafxendi and Patricia Zakreski (eds), *Crafting the Woman Professional in the Long Nineteenth Century* (London 2013) and 'Art and Fashion', Valerie Steele, *Paris Fashion: A Cultural History* (Oxford 1988).

54. 'A Student', 'The Reading Room of the British Museum', Letters to the Editor, *The Times*, 10 May 1862, p.7

55. George Cruikshank, 'Print Room of the British Museum' (1828, V&A: 9544.4)

56. Julia Thomas, *Pictorial Victorians. The Inscription of Values in Word and Image* (Ohio 2004), pp.77–103

57. Holland 1988, p.128

58. Gaudriault 1983, p.102

59. Ibid.

60. Mackrell 1997, p.152

61. Ibid., p.158

62. Diana de Marly, *The History of Haute Couture 1850–1950* (London 1980), p.113

63. Ribeiro 1995, p.3

PLATES

1. Corson 1980, p.228

2. Desmond Hosford, 'The Queen's Hair: Marie-Antoinette, Politics, and DNA', *Eighteenth-Century Studies* (Fall 2004), vol. 38, no. 1, p.189

3. Léon De La Mothe, *Souvenirs sur Marie-Antoinette, Archiduchesse d'Autriche, Reine de France, et sur la Cour de Versailles...* (Paris 1832), vol. 2, p.13

4. Stephens and George 1870–1954, vol. VI, cat. no. 7244

5. Matt Erlin, 'The shaping of Garden Culture in the *Journal Des Luxus Und Der Moden* (1768–1827)', *Publishing Culture and the "Reading Nation": German Book History in the Long Nineteenth Century* (Rochester 2010), p.57

6. *Journal des Luxus und der Moden* (6 January 1791), Jahrgang 6, p.32

7. The eighteenth-century term 'cape' referred to a 'turn-down collar of any size'; Anne Buck, *Dress in Eighteenth-Century England* (London 1979), p.225.

8. Ginsberg 1980, p.28

9. Ibid.

10. Stephens and George 1870–1954, vol. VII, cat. no. 8722

11. 'Fashions for November', *The Times*, 1 December 1807, p.3

12. W.H. Wyatt, *The Lady's Toilette; Containing a Critical Examination of the Nature of Beauty ... An Historical Sketch of the Fashions of France and England, etc.* (London 1808), p.220

13. Charles Baudelaire, *The Painter of Modern Life* (London 2010), p.2. First published 1863 in *Figaro*.

14. Roger-Armand Weigert, *Costumes et Modes d'autrefois: Horace Vernet, Incroyables et merveilleuses Paris 1810–1818* (Paris 1955), p.3

15. *La Belle Assemblée* (1 November 1827), p.218

16. Cumming 2010, p.6

FURTHER READING

Margaret Beetham, *A Magazine of her Own? Domesticity and Desire in the Woman's Magazine 1800–1914* (London 1996)

Dilys Blum, *Illusion and Reality: Fashion in France 1700–1900: The Museum of Fine Arts, Houston, September 10, 1986–January 11, 1987*, exh. cat., The Museum of Fine Arts, Houston, TX (Houston, TX 1986)

Stella Blum (ed.), *Eighteenth-Century French Fashions in Full Colour: 64 Engravings from the 'Galerie des Modes', 1778–1787* (New York 1982)

Richard Corson, *Fashions in Hair: The First Five Thousand Years* (London 1980)

Valerie Cumming, C.W. Cunnington and P.E. Cunnington, *The Dictionary of Fashion History* (Oxford; New York 2010)

Raymond Gaudriault, *La Gravure de mode féminine en france* (Paris 1983)

Charles Harvard Gibbs-Smith, *The Fashionable Lady in the 19th Century* (London 1960)

Madeleine Ginsberg, *An Introduction to Fashion Illustration* (London 1980)

Robert T. Godfrey, *English Caricature, 1620 to the Present: Caricaturists and Satirists – their Art, their Purpose and Influence*, exh. cat., Yale Center for British Art, New Haven, CT; Library of Congress, Washington D.C.; National Gallery of Canada, Ottawa; and Victoria and Albert Museum, London (London 1984)

Avril Hart and Susan North, *Historical Fashion in Detail: The 17th and 18th Centuries* (London 1998)

Vyvyan Beresford Holland, *Hand Coloured Fashion Plates, 1770 to 1889* (London 1988)

Simon Houfe, *The Dictionary of British Book Illustrators and Caricaturists 1800–1914* (Woodbridge 1981)

Lionel Lambourne, *An Introduction to Caricature* (London 1983)

James Laver, Amy De La Haye and Andrew Tucker, *Costume and Fashion: A Concise History* (New York 2002)

James Laver, *17th and 18th Century Costume* (London 1959)

Suzanne Lussier, *Art Deco Fashion* (London 2009)

Alice Mackrell, *An Illustrated History of Fashion: 500 Years of Fashion Illustration* (London 1997)

Constance C. McPhee and Nadine M. Orenstein, *Infinite Jest: Caricature and Satire from Leonardo to Levine*, exh. cat., Metropolitan Museum of Art, New York (New York 2011)

Doris Langley Moore, *Fashion through Fashion Plates, 1771–1970* (New York 1971)

J.L. Nevinson, *Origin and Early History of the Fashion Plate* (Washington, D.C. 1967)

Todd B. Porterfield (ed.), *The Efflorescence of Caricature, 1759–1838* (Farnham; Burlington, VT 2011)

Adelheid Rasche and Gundula Wolter, *Ridikül!: Mode in Der Karikatur, 1600–1900*, exh. cat., Der Kunstbibliothek, Staatliche Museen zu Berlin (Berlin 2003)

Aileen Ribeiro, *Dress and Morality* (New York 1986)

Aileen Ribeiro, *The Art of Dress: Fashion in England and France 1750–1820* (New Haven 1995)

Julian Robinson, *The Golden Age of Style: Art Deco Fashion Illustration* (London 1988)

Frederic George Stephens and Mary Dorothy George, *Catalogue of Political and Personal Satires Preserved in The Department of Prints and Drawings in the British Museum, vols 1–12* (London 1870–1954)

Phyllis G. Tortora and Robert S. Merkel, *Fairchild's Dictionary of Textiles* (New York 1996)

Sarah Grant would like to dedicate this book to her aunt, Margaret Caird, with great love and affection.

Catherine Flood would like to dedicate this book to her mother Maureen Flood, with much love.

ACKNOWLEDGEMENTS

For her patience and dedication in the preparation of this book we would like to thank our very able Editor, Faye Robson. We must also extend sincere thanks to our specialist readers at the Victoria and Albert Museum: Charles Newton, Susan North and Elizabeth Miller.

We gratefully acknowledge the support of Dr Glenn Adamson, Dr Julius Bryant, Mark Eastment, Dr Lesley Miller and Gill Saunders in the realization of this project. For the elegant design of the book we are indebted to the vision of Emily Chicken, of Peepstudio. We were fortunate enough to have valuable assistance with picture research from our curatorial interns, Zenia Malmer and Carys Bailey, and we are grateful to Rowan Bain for her help with object photography.